Enhancing the Abilities of Persons with Alzheimer's and Related Dementias

◆ ◆ ◆ ◆ ◆ ◆ ◆ ◆ ◆ ◆ ◆ ◆ ◆ ◆ ◆

A Nursing Perspective

Pam Dawson, R.N., M.Sc.N., is a Clinical Nurse Specialist in the Department of Extended Care, Sunnybrook Health Sciences Center and is cross appointed to the Faculty of Nursing, University of Toronto, Canada. Her clinical and research interests are in the areas of care for older persons with dementia and their families. Her publications have appeared in *The Canadian Nurse, Geriatric Nursing,* and *The Gerontologist* among other journals. She received her graduate degree from Duke University of Durham, North Carolina.

Donna L. Wells, R.N., M.H.Sc., is an Assistant Professor in the Faculty of Nursing, University of Toronto, Toronto, Ontario, Canada. Her clinical and research interests are in the areas of cognitive impairment and decision making for older persons. Her publications have appeared in *The Canadian Nurse, The Journals of Geriatric Nursing, Gerontological Nursing,* and *Orthopaedic Nursing,* among other journals. She received her M.H.Sc degree from the University of Toronto and is a doctoral candidate at York University in Toronto.

Karen Kline, R.N., M.Sc.N., is a Clinical Nurse Specialist, Acute Care, Lion's Gate Hospital, British Columbia and is cross appointed in the Faculty of Nursing, University of British Columbia in Vancouver. Her clinical and research interests are in the areas of cognitive impairment and behavioral problems in older persons. Her publications have appeared in *Perspectives,* and she has presented workshops across British Columbia. She received her undergraduate and graduate degrees from the University of Toronto.

Enhancing the Abilities of Persons with Alzheimer's and Related Dementias

✦ ✦ ✦ ✦ ✦ ✦ ✦ ✦ ✦ ✦ ✦ ✦ ✦ ✦ ✦ ✦

A Nursing Perspective

Pam Dawson, RN, MScN

Donna L. Wells, RN, MHSc

Karen Kline, RN, MScN

Springer Publishing Company
New York

Springer Publishing Company, Inc.
536 Broadway
New York, NY 10012-3955

    96 97 / 5 4 3

Library of Congress Cataloging-in-Publication Data

Dawson, Pam (Pamela)
    Enhancing the abilities of persons with Alzheimer's and related
dementias: a nursing perspective / Pam Dawson, Donna L. Wells,
Karen Kline.
      p. cm.
    Includes bibliographical references and index.
    ISBN 0-8261-7790-5
     1. Alzheimer's disease—Nursing. 2. Senile dementia—Nursing.
3. Alzheimer's disease—Patients—Care. 4. Senile dementia—
Patients—Care. I. Wells, Donna L. II. Kline, Karen.
III. Title.
    [DNLM: 1. Alzheimer's Disease—nursing. 2. Alzheimer's Disease—
rehabilitation. 3. Dementia, Senile—nursing. 4. Dementia,
Senile—rehabilitation. WM 220 D272e 1993]
RC523.D4 1993
618.97'6831—dc20
DNLM/DLC
for Library of Congress   93-12113
                                             CIP

Printed in the United States of America

This book is dedicated to
Virginia Stone,
a pioneer in the field of
gerontological nursing

CONTENTS

Contents

LIST OF FIGURES

ACKNOWLEDGMENTS

THE AUTHORS WISH TO ACKNOWLEDGE DR. NATHAN HERR-man for his review and editorial assistance of the book, and for his patience. His thoughtful critique has been invaluable to the completion of the book.

We also thank Maribel Lorayes for her assistance in the final typing and preparation of the manuscript, and to Claire Lorayes for the art work. Charlene Boston is to be thanked as well for the typing of earlier versions of the book.

The support and encouragement of Ms. Marilyn MacTavish and Dr. Dorothy Pringle has been greatly appreciated.

To our students and colleagues, Cathy Lyle, Brian Hart, and Dorothy Merner, Randa Hirst, and Susan Dutton, we express our thanks. As well, we have appreciated the willing participation of the residents and nurses at Sunnybrook Health Science Centre in the evolution of this book.

Finally, and most important of all, we wish to express our deeply felt gratitude to our families who faithfully encouraged us, and supported us in our belief that this book would be of help to others.

INTRODUCTION

THIS BOOK IS ABOUT THE NURSING CARE OF OLDER PERSONS WITH ALZHEIMER'S DISEASE. Nurses have long cared for people with dementia. Although we seek to give such care in the most humane way possible, care of demented individuals is very difficult. There is no "cure" to aim for. Communication with the demented individual is frustrating and it is easy for caregivers to lose sight of the human being they are caring for because the possibility for normal human rapport is so diminished.

"Caring and the value of human life are a part of our moral fabric," point out Cohen and Eisdorfer in their book on the experience of Alzheimer's disease. Therefore, by way of introducing our book, the nature of the disease, and our perspective on nursing care, we believe that it is valuable for nurses to imagine how the experience of dementia might feel.

• THE EXPERIENCE OF DEMENTIA AS A JOURNEY •

We imagine that the experience of having Alzheimer's disease might be similar to a journey by train with an unknown destination:

I am going on a long journey by train. As I begin, the city skyscrapers and country landscape look familiar. As I continue my journey, the view reminds me of times gone by and I feel relaxed and comfortable. The other passengers on the train appear to be feeling the same way and I engage in pleasant conversation with them.

As the journey progresses, things begin to look different. The buildings have odd shapes and the trees don't look quite the way I remember them. I know that they are buildings and trees, but something about them is not quite right. Maybe I'm in a different country with different architecture and plant life. It feels a bit strange, even unnerving.

I decide to ask the other passengers about the strangeness I feel, but I notice that they seem unperturbed. They are barely taking notice of the passing scenery. Maybe they have been here before. I ask some questions but nothing seems different to them. I wonder if my mind is playing tricks on me. I decide to act as if everything looks all right, but because it does not, I have to be on my guard. This places some tension on me, but I believe I can tolerate it for the remainder of the trip. I do, however, find myself becoming so preoccupied with appearing all right that my attention is diverted from the passing scenery.

After some time, I look out the window again and this time I know that something is wrong. Everything looks strange and unfamiliar! There is no similarity to anything I can recall from the past. I must do something. I talk to the other passengers about the strangeness I feel. They look dumbfounded and when they answer, they talk in a new language. Why won't they talk in English, I wonder? They look at me knowingly and with sympathy. I've got to get to the bottom of this so I keep after them to tell me where the train is and where it is going. The only answers I get are in this strange language, and even when I talk, my words sound strange to me. Now I am truly frightened.

At this point, I figure that I have to get off this train and find my way home. I had not bargained for this when I started. I get up to leave and bid a pleasant goodbye. I don't get very far, though, as the other passengers stop me and take me back to my seat. It seems they want me to stay on the train whether I want to or not. I try to explain but they just talk in that strange language.

Outside the window, the scenery is getting even more frightening. Strange, inhuman-looking beings peer into the window at me. I decide to make a run for it. The other passengers are not paying much attention to me so I slip out of my seat and quietly walk toward the back of the car. There's a door! It is difficult to push but I must. It begins to open and I push harder. Maybe now I will get away. Even though it looks pretty strange out there I know I will never find my way home if I do not get off that train. I am just ready to jump when hands suddenly appear from nowhere and grab me from behind. I try to get away. I try to fight them off, but I can feel them pulling me back onto the train. I hear the door shut. They take me back to my seat. I realize now that I will never get off this train; I will never get home.

How sad I feel. I did not say goodbye to my friends or children. As far as I know they do not know where I am. The passengers look sympathetic, but they do not know how sad I feel. Maybe if they knew they would let me off the train. I stop smiling, stop eating, stop trying to talk, and avoid looking out the window. The passengers look worried. They force me to eat. It is difficult because I am too sad to be hungry.

I have no choice now. I have to go along with the passengers because they seem to know where the journey will end. Maybe they will get me there safely. I fervently wish that I had never started out on this journey but I know I cannot go back.

The other passengers on the train are meant to be nurses. As nurses, our aim is to assist older persons with dementia to make this journey with as much dignity and comfort as possible.

• DEMENTIA OF THE ALZHEIMER'S TYPE AS A DISEASE •

Dementia of the Alzheimer's type is the most common form of the dementias (Evans et al., 1989; Mortimer & Hutton, 1985), and one of the most pervasive health problems for older persons (Heacock, Walton, Beck & Mercer, 1991). Although the disease primarily involves a progressive mental deterioration, often referred to as "cognitive impairment." it concomitantly affects all aspects of a person's life, including the ability to relate to others and the environment, and the ability to care for oneself (Herrmann, 1991), as reflected in the imaginative train journey. Dementia is a diffuse cortical disorder affecting both hemispheres and causing a global deterioration in function involving the intellect, motor behavior (changes in gait and speech), emotion, personality, perception and judgment, and bodily physiology (Pryse-Phillips & Murray, 1986).

Alzheimer's disease has been found "wherever studies have been conducted in a population with a large enough elderly population" (Brody & Cohen, 1989). In the United States, about 4% to 6% of persons over 65 years of age, and 30% of those over 80, suffer from Alzheimer's disease (Brody & Cohen, 1989). In Canada, 5% to 10% of people aged 65 and over, and 20% of those over 80, suffer from the disease (Herrmann, 1991). Herrmann further reports that these figures are probably underestimated.

The number of individuals with Alzheimer's dementia is anticipated to increase in the next few decades as the population continues to grow older, age being a significant risk factor for the disease (Brody & Cohen, 1989; Evans et al., 1989). The public health impact, given the increasing longevity and rise in the prevalence of the disease, is enormous (Burns & Buckwalter, 1988; Evans et al., 1989). The impact of dementia on caregivers will also intensify as more than 50% of individuals in nursing homes now suffer from dementia (Herrmann, 1991; Reichel, cited in Heacock, Walton, Beck, & Mercer, 1991). The significant burden, however, rests with families who continue to be the major caregivers (Rabins, 1988).

Alzheimer's dementia has been the focus of a great deal of study. Most research has concentrated on the etiology and pathophysiology of the disease, the diagnosis and prediction of its clinical course, and its effect on family caregivers. There is a need for progress to be made to improve the day-to-day situation for individuals affected with Alzheimer's disease and their caregivers, while awaiting breakthroughs in the cause and treatment of the disease (Buckwalter, Abraham, & Neundorfer, 1988; Brody & Cohen, 1989). From a personal point of view, we have felt the need for a more applied focus or specific information that is assistive in caring for individuals with Alzheimer's disease. The purpose of this book is to provide such information, by linking the behaviors of individuals with Alzheimer's dementia to specific features of the disease through a careful study of the general and specific research literature. Through this linkage we derive practical interventions for allowing these individuals to optimize their remaining abilities.

This book grew out of many years of our work as clinical nurse specialists involving the identification of behaviors of individuals with dementia that place unusual demands on caregivers. This led us to the literature for a further description of the behaviors as they derive from and relate to the disease. Our interest focused on gaining an understanding of dementia, its impact on the individual's ability to participate in life's daily activities, and its specific relationship to caregiving activities. With this information, we developed an assessment and caregiving approach for older persons with dementia, which we applied and used in clinical practice, and subsequently refined. What is important about the work is that it synthesizes individual behaviors observed in practice with an understanding of certain features of the disease and applies this information directly to the caregiving process. We assume that those reading our book will have an initial or general understanding of normal aging and of dementia, and will have completed related assessment procedures.

Another distinction of our work is its focus on enhancing the abilities of older persons with Alzheimer's dementia. We believe that this perspective, which we call Enablement, provides a positive attitude in the approach to care, despite the absence of a prevention or cure for this devastating disease. In planning care that is abilities-enhancing, an understanding of how the disease affects the abilities of individuals with dementia is critical. As nurses, we are concerned not too much with the disease per se, but with the person who has to live with the effects of the disease, and the caregivers who provide care. We believe that the human experience continues under Alzheimer's, but with the additional challenges of living with a progressive and pervasive disease. One way to assist the person in meeting these challenges, and to provide continuity in the life experience, is with an approach that enhances the persons's abilities. Although Alzheimer's disease is devastating, this enhancement may provide quality in the life experience. It is our hope that this book will provide knowledge about the abilities of individuals in relation to Alzheimer's disease so that continuity and quality of life can be preserved. We also hope that this information will excite nurses and other caregivers and ease the experience of caregiving.

• ORGANIZATION OF THE BOOK •

Chapter 1 describes the Enablement perspective, our suggested approach to caring for older persons with dementia, and outlines the events that led to the development of this particular approach. Enablement is defined, and an Enablement nursing process, which derives from our definition, is elaborated. A method of moving from the Enablement perspective to actual caregiving practice is detailed. This method is called a content methodology, it provides a way to define content for nursing practice: specifically, nursing assessment and caregiving approaches based on the general and specific research literature. Both Enablement and the Content Methodology Process are illustrated repeatedly throughout the book in the presentation of four areas of human abilities threatened by Alzheimer's disease: social, self-care, interactional, and interpretive abilities.

Chapter 2 focuses on self-care abilities, defined as those discrete abilities underlying the capacity to carry out activities of daily living. The abilities presented for study in relation to particular clinical features of Alzheimer's disease include voluntary movements, spatial orientation, and the use of purposeful movements in carrying out self-care. Drawing from the literature, assessment methods are outlined and nursing actions detailed.

In Chapter 3, the social abilities of individuals, or the abilities to engage in or respond to social cues and to behave normatively in social contexts, are described in relation to Alzheimer's disease. These abilities include the giving and receiving of attention, the use of appropriate behavior in social situations, and principles of communication or conversation. Various, but specific nursing activities or interventions including conversational groups, music, and humor are discussed.

Chapter 4 describes the interactional abilities of older persons who may be threatened with dementia. Language comprehension, expressive abilities, and writing abilities are examined with regard to aphasia, the major clinical feature of dementia that affects language. Methods of determining the individual's language abilities are illustrated. Nursing actions are illustrated, including the formulation of meaningful communication practices and the effective use of reading and writing abilities.

Chapter 5 is devoted to interpretive abilities, or those capacities that allow individuals to derive meaning from the environment. The abilities to recognize self and others, to recognize objects by touch, and to relate to time are included in the discussion. Several strategies for assessment and management of these abilities are considered and examples included.

In Chapter 6 the importance of clinical practice for older persons with Alzheimer's disease that is research-based is summarized, and future directions are charted.

Throughout the book, the pronoun "she" is used when referring to cognitively impaired older persons. The feminine pronoun was selected because the majority of older persons in the population are women, including those with dementia (Brody & Cohen, 1989).

• REFERENCES •

Brody, J. A., & Cohen, D. (1989). Epidemiologic aspects of Alzheimer's disease. *Journal of Aging and Health, 1*(2), 139–149.

Buckwalter, K. C., Abraham, I. L., & Neundorfer, M. M. (1988). Alzheimer's disease: Involving nursing in the development and implementation of health care for patients and families. *Nursing Clinics of North America, 23*((1), 1–9.

Burns, E. M., & Buckwalter, K. C. (1988). Pathophysiology and etiology of Alzheimer's disease. *Nursing Clinics of North America, 23*(1), 11–29.

Cohen, D., & Eisdorfer, C. (1986). *The loss of self.* New York: NAL Penguin.

Evans, D. A., Funkenstein, H. H., Albert, M. S., Scherr, P. A., Cook, N. R., Chown, M. J., Heberrt, L. E., Hennekens, Charles H., & Taylor, J. O. (1989). *Journal of the American Medical Association, 262*(18), 2551–2556.

Heacock, P., Walton, C., Beck, C., & Mercer, S. (1991). Caring for the cognitively impaired: Reconceptualizing disability and rehabilitation. *Journal of Gerontological Nursing, 17*(3), 23–26.

Herrmann, N. (1991). Confusion and dementia in the elderly. In *Mental health and aging* (pp. 35–47). Ottawa, Ontario, Canada: The National Advisory Council on Aging.

Pryse-Phillips, W., & Murray, T. J. (1986). *Essential neurology* (3rd ed.). New York: Medical Examination Publishing Company.

Rabins, P. V. (1988). Psychosocial aspects of dementia. *Journal of Clinical Psychiatry, 49*(5), 29–31.

ONE

CARING FOR OLDER PERSONS WITH DEMENTIA:

THE ENABLEMENT PERSPECTIVE

A FEW YEARS AGO, IN THE PROCESS OF REFLECTING ON OUR caregiving practices, we came to the idea of Enablement as a way to think about our care of cognitively impaired older persons. Although we had been working from a philosophy of rehabilitation for a number of years, with a focus on the person's functional ability rather than cure, we still were not satisfied with our care. The dominant emphasis was on disability. Individuals were seen as not-able, and care sometimes was provided solely at a maintenance level. Moreover, we often observed the phenomenon of excess disability (Dawson, Kline, Wiancko, & Wells, 1986; Dawson & Wells, 1987) defined as impairment in function beyond that which could be accounted for on the basis of the disease (Brody, Kleban, Lawton, & Moss, 1974; Kahn, 1966). We speculated that the presence of excess disability was related to many factors within the purview of nursing. For instance, restlessness or agitation in persons with dementia is often attributed to the disease by health

1

care professionals. The behavior, however, may simply be related to physical discomfort or features within the environment. In relation to these reflections, we asked ourselves a number of questions: (1) How can excess disability be prevented? (2) How can we shift our focus of care from disease and disability to an abilities focus? (3) How can the lives of individuals with dementia be made meaningful? and finally, (4) What is it that characterizes, or makes distinctive, the nursing care of individuals suffering from dementia? Emerging from our earlier work (Dawson, Kline, Wiancko, & Wells, 1986), the idea of Enablement, *focuses attention on the person's abilities or resources*, came to mind as a possible way of addressing these questions.

We believe that Enablement, as an approach to nursing care, can foster meaningful life experiences for individuals despite the presence of cognitive impairment. We also propose that a focus on abilities permits both continuity in life experiences and a sense of personal competence.

Enablement offers a perspective which emphasizes the person's capacity to engage as fully as possible in day-to-day living, thus facilitating the individual's journey through the unexpected experience of dementia. Enabling others through life transitions and unfamiliar events has been identified as one of several processes of caring in the practice of nursing (Swanson, 1991). Caring has long been considered central to nursing practice (Benner & Wrubel, 1989; Leininger, 1981, 1988; Morse, Bottorff, Neander, & Solberg, 1991; Watson, 1988). Swanson's findings suggest that "an enabling caregiver is one who uses his or her expert knowledge to the betterment of the other. The purpose of enabling is to facilitate the other's capacity to grow, heal, and/or practice self-care" (p. 164).

Enablement, which requires a focus on abilities, may also serve to counter the dominance of the biomedical approach to persons with dementia, with its focus on body and mind pathology and expectations of incompetence (Lyman, 1989). The biomedical model of care has been noted to lead to the objectification of the patient (Berdes, 1987). Within this model, patients are seen as inanimate objects—as a disease—and consequently, as passive recipients of care. A nihilistic, "nothing can be done" orientation may also arise.

Using the idea of enablement as a conceptual guide to nursing practice provides a way to develop substantive knowledge for the discipline, a challenge offered to nurses by Meleis (1991). The use of a conceptual approach like Enablement focuses the conduct and interpretation of theory and research (in either prior or prospective works) specifically on nursing concerns, such as the human response to disease. In the case of dementia, the nursing interest is in elaborating the influence of dementia on discrete human capacities to partake in day-to day living, and in specifying precise enabling caregiving activities. This reflects a distinctive focus of nursing; the search for knowledge and understanding of human beings' responses to health and illness, in order to offer meaningful care or to help the individual care for the self (Meleis, 1991). This knowledge can be articulated easily to others by nurses, hence serving pedagogical purposes, or the function of explaining to others what nurses do and what the discipline is about.

• *WHAT IS ENABLEMENT?* •

Our working definition of Enablement is "the process of going into abilities." This definition derives from synthesizing and adapting the dictionary definitions of en-, able, and -ment (Webster's Ninth New Collegiate Dictionary, 1987):

en-   meaning: to put into . . .,
able   meaning: marked by intelligence, knowledge, skill, or competence, and,
-ment   meaning: action: process; state or condition resulting from (a specified action)

Proceeding from this definition, Enablement involves assisting the other to use her abilities or resources. This constitutes a shift from the traditional preoccupation with the disease, its pathology and related disabilities.

Using Enablement as our perspective, we have elaborated the Enablement nursing process which is depicted in Figure 1.1. Applied to caregiving practices, the Enablement Nursing Process constitutes a course of action taken by the nurse to provide the opportunity for individuals to engage in the daily course of living according to their abilities. This course of action is guided by an in-depth knowledge of the disease. As Dawson (1987) has noted, to provide knowledgeable and personalized care which is enabling for older persons with cognitive impairment, it is necessary to have knowledge about Alzheimer's disease and to interpret this information specifically in the context of nursing practice goals. Enablement orients the nursing study and interpretation of the disease to an understanding of its effect on the individual's ability to engage in daily life experiences. The disease is not studied for diagnostic or treatment purposes. Instead, it is studied to determine how its clinical features, that is, the signs and symptoms associated with the pathology of the disease, affect particular human abilities to carry out day-to-day life activities. We know that the abilities of individuals experiencing a dementia such as Alzheimer's disease can be affected in a number of pervasive and discrete ways. If nurses can identify and promote retained abilities and/or compensate for lost abilities, they can enable the individual in the life experience, and excess disability may be prevented.

Within the Enablement Nursing Process, the nursing assessment is intended to purposefully elicit retained or remaining abilities and/or those abilities which are at risk of decline or loss as a result of the disease process. The four areas of abilities that we have identified as necessary for day-to-day living are self-care, social, interactional and interpretive abilities (Dawson, Kline, Wiancko, & Wells, 1986). Our concern is with the discrete abilities that underlie an individual's capacity to engage in living, rather than the larger categories of activities of daily living, such as bathing and grooming.

In order to elicit the discrete abilities of individuals with dementia in these four areas, nursing assessment approaches are as

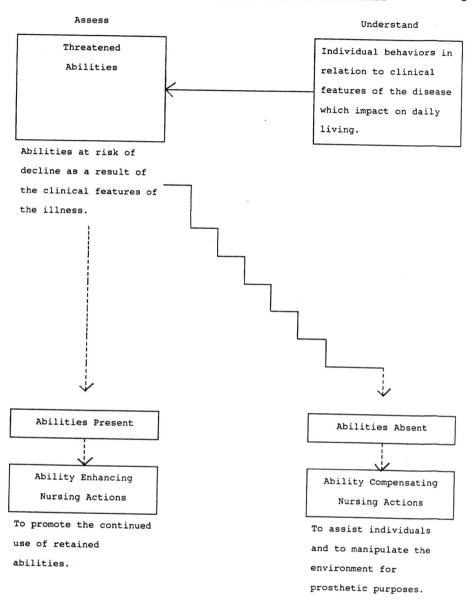

Figure 1.1
The Enablement Nursing Process constitutes a course of action taken by the nurse to provide the opportunity for individuals to engage in the daily course of living according to their abilities.

follows. We begin with the assessment of simple abilities. Then we proceed to the assessment of those abilities that are more complex, on the assumption that simple abilities are easier to carry out. Our clinical experience and the literature further suggests that self-care and social abilities are familiar and overlearned, and remain longer than the more abstract interactional and interpretive abilities. Therefore, self-care and social abilities are elicited first, followed by an assessment of interactional and interpretive abilities. Our precise assessment methods have evolved from a study of the research on Alzheimer's disease and related disorders.

When abilities are found to be retained or present, then *ability-enhancing* nursing actions are designed and offered. These actions may derive from suggestions in the research, from experience, or from the creativity and imagination of the nurse. The intent is to promote the continued use of retained abilities. The opportunity to use one's remaining abilities facilitates participation and continuity in daily living, and fosters a sense of personal mastery.

Ability-enhancing nursing actions are offered initially even when assessment suggests that abilities are lost. We do this because the ability may simply be dormant as a consequence of disuse or excess disability. When ability-enhancing nursing activities remain ineffective and the assessment findings continue to indicate that abilities are lost, then *ability-compensating nursing actions* are provided. These nursing activities create the possibility for the person to maintain continuity in daily living events. Ability-compensating nursing actions may be designed to assist individuals in a particular activity, or to manipulate the environment for supportive purposes.

In one of our educational sessions for the nurses, we employ the following vignette to illustrate the Enablement Nursing Process.

A daughter who is caring for her father at home leaves him a note to turn off the stove when the clock bell rings. The father reads this note in her presence. But he seems to "ignore" the reminder, as she finds the oven on when she returns home despite her observation that the bell has indeed rung. The father's behavior, if not understood, could be interpreted as a lack of motivation or cooperation, or disinterest. This may not be the case.

Aphasia is one of the clinical feature of dementia underlying the father's behavior. The ability to process or understand written information may be affected. This means that although an individual is able to read, he may read without comprehension of what has been read, and therefore, cannot follow through. In this vignette, the father's behavior—reading without follow-through—was a consequence of the lost ability to understand written communication. Hence, he could not act on his daughter's note.

Two distinct abilities require assessment: reading ability and reading comprehension. The method of assessing each ability is described later in this book. When the ability to follow through on what has been read is lost, as in the father's experience, written memory aids will not be helpful and can in fact be a source of stress. The daughter will need to perform the task herself, or compensate by making a telephone call at an appropriate time to relay the message. Despite the loss of reading comprehension, it is important to encourage the father to continue to read to enhance his reading ability and to help him retain a sense of competence. Even though the individual does not understand what is read, the activity of reading can be a source of satisfaction. In the book *Memory Board* (Ruhl, 1987), an older woman with a diagnosis of Alzheimer's disease reads aloud to a blind man. Not only is the woman able to continue to practice the ability to read, she is also able to help another human being.

For nurses, the Enablement perspective orients the study and care of individuals with cognitive impairment toward a focus on human abilities. It further incorporates a knowledge of the clinical and behavioral features of dementia, thereby offering a systematic, research-based guide to practice.

• *ENABLEMENT AND EXCESS DISABILITY* •

Careful attention to the abilities of cognitively impaired individuals may help to prevent or reverse excess disability. This prevention or reversal is an explicit objective within the conceptual approach of Enablement and in nursing practice. Salisbury (1991) presents an excellent review and discussion of the relevance of excess disability as a key concept in gerontological nursing.

Excess disability may arise in individuals with cognitive impairment through the disuse of existing abilities. Individuals who are not mobilized on a regular and frequent basis may develop excess flexion (see Figure 1.2). Excess disability can arise following acute physical or psychological disease. Excess disability in this case is a consequence of professionals failure to determine the premorbid level of ability and setting this level as the outcome goal. The presenting state in the unfolding of the disease is accepted as the actual level of ability, rather than excess disability. Some individual behaviors may be attributed to the disease when in fact they derive from another more benign source that is reversible. For example, restlessness or agitation often occurs in relation to constipation or from the use of physical and chemical restraint. In these instances the behavior is not to be assigned to the disease process and left unexamined, but rather investigated and remediated. Excess disability may be a result of inappropriate stimulation in the environment (Dawson, Kline, Wiancko, & Wells, 1986; Hiatt, 1987). When existing abilities are recorded as part of the Enablement Nursing Process and nursing activities are ability-enhancing, excess disability may be recognized, prevented or reversed.

• ENABLEMENT AND ENVIRONMENTAL PRESS •

The focus on human abilities also requires a consideration of the environment in which the individual lives. Roberts and Algase (1988) note that consideration of environment is essential to an understanding of the functioning and care of older persons, and even more so for those persons with Alzheimer's disease.

The environment or milieu is known to affect the behavior of individuals with cognitive impairment (Hall & Buckwalter, 1987; Hiatt, 1987; Skolaski-Pellitteri, 1983). The concern with human-

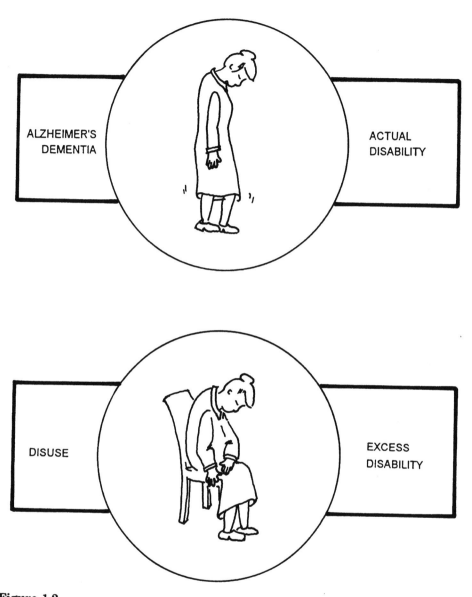

Figure 1.2
Actual disability is the disability associated with the disease, whereas excess diability is not a result of the disease. It arises from the disuse of remaining abilities.

environment interaction has been central to the nursing profession since Florence Nightingale first described nursing as optimizing the environment to promote health and healing (Meleis, 1991). Meleis suggests that most clinicians "pay lip service to it." In the Enablement model of care, environment is integral to nursing's practice, and cannot be ignored.

The concept of environmental press, developed by Lawton and Nahemow (1973) and adapted for our purposes, is helpful in understanding the potential effect of the environment on the behavior and abilities of individuals with cognitive impairment. According to Lawton and Nahemow, environmental press refers to any stimulation in the environment. Hiatt (1987) points out several sources of potential environmental stimulation:

1 the physical features of the environment, such as sights, light, sounds, textures, temperature, smells, and space itself;
2 the social environment, meaning the number of persons occupying a space, their activities, and relationships with one another;
3 environmental norms of expectations and policies.

The noise of radios or televisions, heat or cold, disorganized or catastrophic reaction of others with cognitive impairment, crowding, restrictive institutional policies, unfamiliar procedures, or objects increase the press in the environment of the older person with cognitive impairment. Lawton and Nahemow maintain that the individual's ability to manage the stimulation or press in the environment is related to her competence and behavior.

There is an important relationship between the competence of the individual and stimulation in the environment. When an individual's competence is low, then less environmental stimulation can be tolerated by that individual (see Figure 1.3). An individual with cognitive impairment may be easily burdened by excessive or inappropriate stimulation and respond behaviorally by becoming agitated or withdrawing. The behavior of the individual should not be attributed to the disease or some personal characteristic but to the environment.

When individual competence is high and environmental stimulation is low, the individual may be underchallenged and react by creating her own stimulation (see Figure 1.4). At times, these reactions, such as shouting, may be unpleasant or seem inappropriate. It is important to interpret these behaviors with respect to an impoverished environment, rather than to personal characteristics or the disease.

The Enablement perspective, with its focus on human abilities, helps to describe the competence of the individual. When stimulation in the environment is appraised with the individual's abilities in mind, congruence between abilities and environmental stimuli may be achieved. Lawton (1970) points out that a prosthetic environment offers assistance for all aspects of a person's functioning and support for the person's sense of personal effectiveness.

The ideas of Enablement, excess disability, and environmental press are extremely useful in caring for persons with cognitive impairment. The focus on abilities in relation to the disease experience potentially reduces the risk of cognitively impaired individuals acquiring excess disability. Knowledge of an individual's competencies helps us to make decisions about appropriate environmental stimulation, and when environment and human competence are congruent, excess disability may be prevented.

• ENABLEMENT AND CONTENT FOR NURSING PRACTICE •

How do we move from the idea of Enablement to actual caregiving practices? Again, some questions are instructive. Thinking back to the enabling caregiver, what is the expert knowledge that nurses can use to the betterment of the other? How do we derive this expert knowledge? How do we come to know about human resources or abilities in the face of cognitive impairment so that we can facilitate the person's capacity to grow, heal and/or practice self care, or help to preserve some continuity in the life experience?

We have developed a method to examine and interpret the litera-

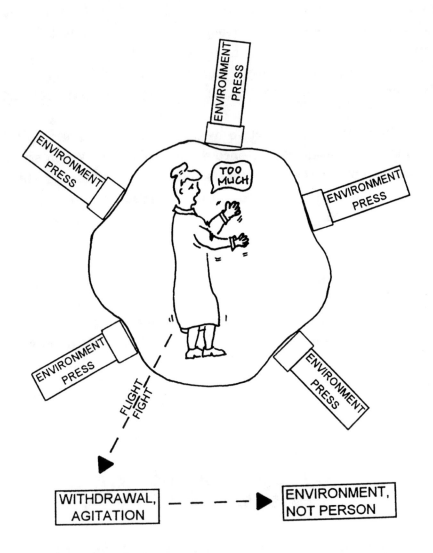

Figure 1.3
High environmental press refers to stimulation in the environment that exceeds
the competence of the individual.

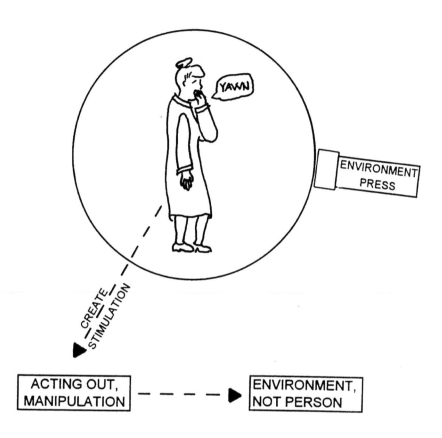

Figure 1.4
Low environment press refers to stimulation in the environment that is below the competence of the individual.

ture for the explicit purpose of defining expert knowledge and practice content (Dawson & Wells, 1992; Dawson, Kline, Wiancko & Wells, 1986; Dawson, 1987; Wells, 1983, 1985, 1987). The process, called a "Content Methodology," is a rigorous procedure which is consistent with our perspective of Enablement. It is a method of deriving enablement-relevant research and information from the literature by "dissecting" each Alzheimer's symptom into its component parts. It is useful in bridging the gap between our conceptual approach of Enablement, the research findings, and nursing practice.

Content Methodology helps in arriving at a substantive base for nursing practice for individuals with dementia. While the dementia research literature is vast, it has been concerned mainly with uncovering the etiology of the disease, defining caregiver burden, and developing measures of cognitive function. The latter is mostly useful for determining disease diagnosis, its severity and treatment. This literature is not immediately useful in understanding how cognitive impairment affects the person's ability to engage in discrete activities of daily living, or in deciding which nursing activities are most appropriate. With some notable exceptions (e.g., Beck & Heacock, 1988; Levy, 1987), we have found that the nursing literature in the area of dementia fails to tie together assessment and caregiving activities with individual behaviors observed in practice, research findings, and a conceptual orientation. The nursing actions suggested are often general versus specific in nature, and nursing practice consequently lacks specificity. We believe that this absence of specificity in practice affects both the individual's care and the contribution of meaningful information by nurses to intra- and interprofessional discussions.

The purpose of the Content Methodology procedure is to define practice content in relation to phenomena of interest to nurses, and for which little specific substantive nursing literature exists regarding caregiving. In this instance, we are interested in understanding how the clinical features of dementia impact on the individual's ability to socialize, perform self-care, interact with, and interpret

1. Behaviors of individuals requiring mediation by caregivers are identified through:
   (a) clinical observation,
   (b) a knowledge of the general literature.
2. An explanation of the behavior(s) is sought with reference to the clinical feature(s) of the disease. This knowledge is acquired through a study of the general literature.
3. The specific research (when available) regarding the behavior of interest and the related clinical feature(s) of the disease is studied with regard to:
   (a) threatened abilities,
   (b) methods of assessment.
4. Nursing approaches are designed to maintain existing abilities or compensate for a loss of abilities.

Figure 1.5
The Content Methodology Process is a method of examining and interpreting the literature for the explicit purpose of defining expert knowledge and practice content.

others and the environment. From this understanding, we have developed a nursing assessment instrument and caregiving approaches that assist individuals with Alzheimer's dementia in their day-to-day living[1].

• ELABORATION OF THE CONTENT METHODOLOGY PROCESS •

The Content Methodology procedure involves an iterative process of moving between clinical practice and the literature (see Figure 1.5). It begins by noting the behaviors of individuals that require mediation by caregivers, either observed in practice or encountered in a general reading of the literature.

To further understand individual behaviors as they might derive from or relate to the phenomenon of interest, such as dementia, a rereading of the general literature is conducted. This literature may inform us, for example, that elders with cognitive impairment expe-

[1]The nursing assessment instrument is included in the Appendix. It may be referred to throughout the book as we describe methods of assessment in each of the four areas of abilities.

rience difficulty with language and communication. But knowing this offers little precise direction for communicating with these individuals. Therefore, it becomes necessary to identify and explain those discrete elements of language dysfunction that elders with dementia may experience. This requires a reading of the more specific research literature, when and where such literature exists.

The specific research is studied and interpreted with regard to the impact of the particular clinical feature(s) of the disease on an individual's ability to perform daily living activities. The intent is to identify those discrete abilities, or other resources of the individual, that may be threatened in the presence of the clinical feature. The focus on abilities of the person follows from the nursing perspective of Enablement that we have previously elaborated.

Assessment methods from the research are then scrutinized to decide if they can be adapted to elicit the abilities or resources in question. If not, assessment methods are created. Individuals can then be assessed to determine the presence or absence of abilities or other human resources.

Nursing approaches are developed based on assessment findings, using any caregiving insights gleaned from the literature and/or from experience. These approaches are intended either to maintain abilities which remain, or to compensate for a loss of abilities.

Through the Content Methodology process, a nursing assessment and caregiving framework has evolved for older persons with dementia. This process is illustrated repeatedly in the remainder of this book. We believe that this framework offers specificity for practice, enhancing the expertise and depth of each nurse's practice to the betterment of individuals receiving our care.

• REFERENCES •

Beck, C., & Heacock, P. (1988). Nursing interventions for patients with Alzheimer's disease. *Nursing Clinics of North America, 23*(1), 95–124.
Benner, P., & Wrubel, J. (1989). *The primacy of caring.* Menlo Park, CA: Addison-Wesley.

Berdes, C. (1987). The modest proposal nursing home: Dehumanizing characteristics of nursing homes in memoirs of nursing home residents. *The Journal of Applied Gerontology, 6*(4), 372–388.

Brody, E. M., Kleban, M. H., Lawton, M. P., & Moss, M. (1974). A longitudinal look at excess disabilities in the mentally impaired aged. *Journal of Gerontology, 29,* 79–84.

Dawson, P., Kline, K., Wiancko, D., & Wells, D. (1986). Preventing excess disability in patients with Alzheimer's disease. *Geriatric Nursing, 7*(6), 298–301.

Dawson, P., & Wells, D. (1992). A content methodology for advancing gerontological nursing practice. *Clinical Nurse Specialist, 6*(2), 85–88.

Dawson, P., & Wells, D. (1987). Identifying and reducing excess disability and vulnerability in geriatric patients Part 1 and Part 2. *Canadian Geriatric Medicine Quarterly, 3,* 60–63, 75–77.

Dawson, P. (1987). Cognitive psychopathology and the phenomenon of wandering: Research and clinical nursing approaches. In H. J. Altman (Ed.), *Alzheimer's disease: Problems, prospects, and perspectives* (pp. 249–750). New York: Plenum Press.

Hall, G. R., & Buckwalter, K. C. (1987). Progressively lowered stress threshold: A conceptual model for care of adults with Alzheimer's disease. *Archives of Psychiatric Nursing, 1*(6), 399–406.

Hiatt, L. G. (1987). Environmental design and mentally impaired older people. In H. J. Altman (Ed.), *Alzheimer's disease: Problems, prospects, and perspectives* (pp. 309–320). New York: Plenum Press.

Kahn, R. L. (1965). Comments. In *Mental impairment in the aged.* In M. P. Lawton & F. G. Lawton (Eds.), *Philadelphia Geriatric Center* (pp. 109–114). Philadelphia:

Lawton, M. P. (1970). Assessment, integration and environments for older people. *The Gerontologist, 10,* 38–46.

Lawton, M. P., & Nahemow, L. (1973). Ecology and the aging process. In C. Eisdorfer & M. P. Lawton (Eds.), *The psychology of adult development and aging* (pp. 619–674). Washington: American Psychological Association.

Leininger, M. M. (1988). Leininger's theory of nursing: Cultural care diversity and universality. *Nursing Science Quarterly, 1*(14), 175–181.

Leininger, M. M. (1981). The phenomenon of caring: Importance, research questions, and theoretical considerations. In M.M. Leininger (Ed.), *Caring: An essential human need* (pp. 3–15). Thorofare, NJ: Charles B. Slack.

Levy, L. L. (1987). Psychological intervention and dementia, part II: The cognitive disability perspective. *Occupational Therapy in Mental Health, 7*(4), 13–36.

Lyman, K. A. (1989). Bringing the social back in: A critique of the biomedicalization of dementia. *The Gerontologist, 29*(5), 597–606.

Meleis, A. I. (1991). *Theoretical nursing: Development and progress* (2d ed.). Philadelphia: J.B. Lippincott.

Morse, J. M., Bottorff, J., Neander, W., & Solberg, S. (1991). Comparative analysis of conceptualizations and theories of caring. *Journal of Nursing Scholarship, 23*(2), 119–126.

Roberts, B., & Algase, D. L. (1988). Victims of Alzheimer's disease and the environment. *Nursing Clinics of North America, 23*(1), 83–93.

Ruhl, J. (1987). *Memory board.* Tallahassee, Florida: Naiad Press.

Salisbury, S. A. (1991). Preventing excess disability. In W. C. Chenitz, J. T. Stone, & S. A. Salisbury (Eds.), *Clinical gerontological nursing* (pp. 391–401). Philadelphia: W.B. Saunders.

Skolaski-Pellitteri, T. (1983). Environmental adaptations which compensate for dementia. *Physical and Occupational Therapy in Geriatrics, 3*(1), 31–44.

Swanson, K. M. (1991). Empirical development of a middle range theory of caring. *Nursing Research, 40*(3), 161–166.

Watson, J. (1988). New dimensions of human caring theory. *Nursing Science Quarterly, 1*(4), 175–181.

Webster's Ninth New Collegiate Dictionary. (1987). Springfield, MA: Merriam-Webster.

Wells, D. L. (1987). A systematic approach to the nursing care of acutely ill geriatric patients with cognitive impairment. In H. J. Altman (Ed.), *Alzheimer's disease: Problems, prospects, and perspectives* (pp. 225–233). New York: Plenum Press.

Wells, D. L. (1983). Learning to cope with the hospitalized Alzheimer's patient. *Perspectives, 7*(2), 1–4.

Wells, D. L. (1985). The elderly orthopaedic patient with Alzheimer's disease. *Orthopaedic Nursing, 4*(6), 16–22.

TWO

SELF-CARE ABILITIES

E VENTUALLY, DEMENTIA AFFECTS THE ABILITY TO CARE FOR oneself in basic daily living activities. Self-care abilities are those abilities underlying the capacity to carry out basic functions of daily living, including bathing, grooming, dressing, and safely moving about in the environment. Self-care abilities are learned early in life and are reinforced throughout the lifespan. These abilities may be retained, in part or in whole, even when the person suffers from a progressive, and irreversible dementia. Reisberg (cited in Miller, 1990) notes that the abilities required to perform activities of daily living are preserved until the moderate or more severe stages of the disease. On the other hand, cognitive skills and competency in life tasks deteriorate at different rates in different people (Cohen, Kennedy, & Eisdorfer, cited in Miller, 1990, p. 552), as we have found caring for a large number of people with Alzheimer's disease during the past decade. Supporting our clinical observation, Reed, Jagust, and Seab (1989) found that mental status did not predict ability to perform activities of daily living regardless of the severity of the disease. Therefore, self-care abilities of individuals with dementia should be assessed throughout the course of the disease in order to prevent excess disability in self care.

An additional and important benefit of an abilities-focused approach is that it can offset the tendency of caregivers to encourage dependency behaviors in older persons with cognitive impairment (Barton, Baltes, & Orzech, 1980). These dependency behaviors have the potential to prematurely increase the caregiver burden.

Our approach to the study of self-care abilities differs from traditional approaches that concentrate on defining the more global aspects of daily living activities. A number of discrete abilities or skills are intrinsic to the individual's capacity to carry out basic living activities rendering these skills enormously complex (Briggs, 1990; Weaverdyck, 1987). Our focus is on the recognition and assessment of these discrete abilities. With respect to bathing, we are interested in the individual's ability to extend the arm in combination with other distinct abilities: the initiation, sequencing, completion, and stopping of self-care acts. Typically, conventional measures of self-care abilities are interested in broad levels of dependency. They tend to be disability-oriented, for example, the Index of ADL (Katz, Ford, Moskowitz, Jackson & Jaffe, 1963); the Barthel Self-Care Index (Mahoney & Barthel, 1965); and the Performance Test of ADL (Kuriansky & Gurland, 1976). Beck (1988) explains that instruments to measure daily living functions were developed as a way to assess physical capacities and disabilities, and not to link particular self-care abilities to cognitive deficits; hence, they have not been assistive to actual caregiving. The conceptual perspective of Enablement, combined with the Content Methodology process described in Chapter One, explicitly ties nursing assessment and caregiving strategies to particular cognitive deficits associated with dementia. Most importantly, these approaches focus caregiving attention on the preservation or compensation of abilities.

The specific self-care abilities discussed in this chapter which are affected by Alzheimer's disease are voluntary movements, spatial orientation, and purposeful movements. The related clinical features associated with the disease are, respectively, the development of primitive reflexes and paratonia, spatial disorientation, ideomotor and ideational apraxia, and perseveration. This chapter describes each of these abilities and related clinical features of the disease, along with our specific assessment and nursing approaches.

• *VOLUNTARY MOVEMENTS* •

CLINICAL FEATURES AND THREATENED ABILITIES

Sometimes older people with dementia appear to resist our caregiving. When we attempt to provide bathing, the person may respond by tensing her arms and legs and clutching the nearest object. During mealtime, food may be resisted because the lips are clamped together. This is very disturbing as the nurse is unable to provide sufficient intake. How can these behaviors be interpreted in light of the disease?

It is known that voluntary movement of body parts, including the limbs, fingers and lips, may be affected in Alzheimer's disease by the development of primitive neurological reflexes, such as paratonia, the suck and grasp reflexes (Bakchine, Lacomblez, Palisson, Laurent, & Derouesne, 1989; Tweedy et al., 1982; Villeneuve, Turcotte, Bouchard, Cote, & Jus, 1974). Paratonia, also called hypertonia or the gegenhalten response, refers to muscle resistance to the passive stretch of the limb (Pryse-Phillips & Murray, 1986). It is neurological in origin, involving muscle flexion in response to an assisted movement of extension. Paratonia may be observed when the nurse attempts to straighten the arm or leg for bathing purposes (assisted extension), but finds that the person responds by tensing or bending the limb (flexion). The point is that the individual is not resisting care, but rather is responding involuntarily to a stimulus.

The suck reflex refers to a pursing of the lips in response to a stroking of the lips (Pryse-Phillips & Murray, 1986). In clinical practice, this behavior may be observed during mealtime. When attempting to feed someone with a spoon, the person's lips may close before or while the spoon is being placed into the mouth. The temptation may be to interpret this behavior as resistance to food, when it is in fact an involuntary, neurological reaction to stimulus of the lips.

The grasp reflex is the involuntary grasping of the examiner's hand after the palm of the hand has been lightly stroked and when asked not to (Tweedy et al., 1982). This means that the fingers of the hand will bend or flex when the palm is touched. During hand washing, when a nurse attempts to remove the facecloth from the older person's hand, the washcloth may be grasped more tightly. This involuntary neurological response may be misinterpreted as uncooperative behavior.

Bakchine, Lacomblez, Palisson, Laurent, and Derouesne (1989) examined 91 institutionalized individuals (6 men and 85 women) with dementia of the Alzheimer's type. Neurological examination was undertaken to search for primitive reflexes (among other neurological signs) following procedures developed by Tweedy et al. They found an increasing number of primitive responses, including the suck and the grasp, as cognitive impairment worsened measured by scores on the Mini-Mental State Examination. This finding is similar to Tweedy et al., who assessed 32 older men and women with dementia for the presence of a number of primitive reflexes. Paratonia was not associated with impaired performance on cognitive tests (Tweedy et al., 1982).

The clinical signs of paratonia and the suck and grasp reflexes are not necessary clinical markers of Alzheimer's dementia. Although the clinical signs of suck and grasp reflexes are commonly present in persons with the disease, they may also arise in other diseases and in non-demented aged people. Hence, primitive neurological reflexes are not of medical diagnostic value. Nevertheless, their presence is *always* significant for nursing care, as these neurological reflexes, when present, may interfere with the person's voluntary movement abilities, as explained above. Caregiving strategies will then have to be modified.

Method of Assessment

Individuals with cognitive impairment usually attempt to engage in activities of daily living. To facilitate this participation, it is useful to determine if specific voluntary movement abilities such as lip relaxation, finger extension, and limb extension are retained. If so, these discrete abilities, important in eating, hygiene and grooming activities, can be encouraged and preserved.

The ability of voluntary movement of the lips is assessed by asking the individual to maintain relaxation of the lips when light pressure in the form of a tongue blade or flexed finger is moved along the lips. Voluntary movement ability of the fingers without flexion is determined by requesting the individual to maintain finger extension when the palm of the open hand is gently stimulated or stroked by the examiner's finger. The ability to voluntarily move the limbs without resistance is tested by passively flexing and extending the person's arm or leg each of 4 times to the same degree. When the individual is able to perform these movements voluntarily, these abilities are present.

Nursing Actions

Ability Enhancing

If voluntary movement abilities are present, as is the case with the majority of persons with Alzheimer's disease, then

1. hygiene, grooming and eating activities can be undertaken as commonly performed;
2. passive and active range of motion is undertaken to preserve muscle strength;
3. persons are involved in exercise programs.

When voluntary movements of the limbs are preserved, then bathing and dressing activities can proceed as follows. First, the extremities, then the trunk of the body can be bathed. Dressing and eating can proceed according to the usual routine.

It has been found that reduction in mobility may be related to institutionalization and other excess disabilities or pathologies, rather than to dementia (Pendergast, Calkins, Fisher, & Vickers, 1987; MacLennan, Ballinger, McHarg & Ogston, 1987). Encouraging both range-of-motion exercises and participation in daily exercise routines to preserve muscle tone and strength is therefore critical unless contraindicated. Both are important also for general well being. These activities are undertaken when the ability to voluntarily move the fingers and limbs is preserved.

When the ability to voluntarily move the lips is present, then oral hygiene and nutritional activities do not require modification (provided other abilities, such as swallowing, are preserved). Beck (1988) stresses the importance of oral hygiene in older persons with cognitive impairment both for reasons of general comfort and to promote appetite. It would be useful to encourage the person to perform oral care on their own, as well. Food and fluids may be introduced without as much concern when the person maintains the ability to voluntarily move the lips. To foster adequate nutritional intake and independence in feeding, gentle stroking of the forearm combined with instructions are ability enhancing (Eaton, Mitchell-Bonair, & Friedmann, 1986).

NURSING ACTIONS

Ability Compensating

When the ability for voluntary movement is lost,

1. the method of conducting basic living activities is altered.
2. prosthetic approaches to facilitate oral hygiene and nutritional intake are employed.

For individuals who have lost the ability to voluntarily move their arms and legs, self-care may be facilitated by having the person sit at the side of the bed or at the sink so that gravity can assist the individual in achieving limb extension. A period of time may be required for limb extension to occur. When assisting with bathing, another enabling strategy is to wash the limbs at the end of the bath, so that they do not contract prematurely from stimulation thus causing unnecessary frustration for the caregiver. For placement of a shirt or dress, it is helpful to have the individual in a standing position with the arms in extension. Shirts, blouses, and dresses with closures at the back are desirable. By keeping the arms in extension, back closures can be completed even if the stimulation elicits paratonia. When ambulating the individual, support at the waist rather than the arms to prevent involuntary flexion of the arms during walking, which may offset balance.

When the ability to maintain finger extension is lost, the offsetting goal of practice is to avoid the sequelae of contractures by detering the prolonged grasping of objects. Alternate strategies than range-of-motion, or exercise classes to encourage muscle tone and strength of the fingers and limbs may be necessary. Exercises that do not stimulate paratonia and the grasp reflex are designed; for example, "follow the leader", or throwing a large ball and simply standing. To facilitate bathing the hands, they can be left until the end of the bath. When assisting with dressing, offer one-step instructions such as "relax your fingers," and stand the person, if possible, to prosthetically use gravitational force to extend the fingers to ease putting on shirts, dresses, sweaters and jackets. Avoid the tendency of the person to grasp or clutch objects through planned caregiving that minimizes elicitation of this reflex.

When the ability to relax the lips voluntarily is absent, a straw may be used to facilitate fluid intake as it will stimulate sucking. Paradoxically, the grasp reflex may be considered useful, and can be called upon to facilitate clutching of eating utensils at mealtime. Verbal guidance, such as "open your mouth" spoken before the utensil touches the lips, may also facilitate intake of food at mealtime. Touch may be combined with this measure to promote food intake (Eaton, Mitchell-Bonair, & Friedman, 1986). For safety purposes, only safe, edible objects are placed in the individual's environment.

• *SPATIAL ORIENTATION* •

CLINICAL FEATURES AND THREATENED ABILITIES

The abilities to relate to one's body parts and/or to those of others, and to finding one's way, are spatial orientation abilities. They permit involvement in basic living activities and safe exploration of the environment. One clinical feature of dementia is spatial disorientation. This refers to dysfunction in determining the relationship of one's body parts or body to self, to others, and/or the environment (Liu, Gauthier, & Gauthier, 1991). This entails difficulty in moving or travelling to destinations within the environment and locating one's own or someone else's body parts. Both activities are taken for granted, and yet they are basic for our safety. Beck (1988) points out that safety has been identified as a significant need of the individual with Alzheimer's disease. In the day-to-day living experience of the individual, both the ability to identify specific body parts and the ability to return to a point of origin safely may be compromised in the presence of spatial disorientation. When the ability to determine spatial orientation is affected, numerous implications arise for conducting the activities of hygiene, dressing, grooming, and safe mobilization.

Spatial orientation in terms of the ability to return to a point of origin safely is implicated in dementia when the phenomenon of wandering arises. It is not uncommon in practice to encounter elders with Alzheimer's disease who wander or lose their way. Hussian (1981) defines "wandering" as any change in physical location which results in a person's inability to return to the point of origin with or without prosthetic devices.

Two possible explanations that might account for wandering behavior are the nature of the disease and the environment. First, there may be parietal lobe involvement with dementia. Secondly, any change in perception of the environment or relocation may affect the person's spatial orientation.

Studies have explored both these reasons for the occurrence of wandering behavior. DeLeon, Potegal, and Gurland (1984) administered a series of parietal lobe tests to 21 nursing home residents with a presumed diagnosis of dementia of the Alzheimer's type. Five of the residents were wanderers and 16 were nonwanderers. The wanderers performed less well on the parietal lobe tests. One parietal test included an examination of the ability to discriminate body parts, called a test of right/left orientation. This included successfully following the examiner's commands for identification of one's own and the examiner's body parts, and imitating the hand positions as modelled by the examiner. Right/left orientation, or the spatial ability regarding the identification of body parts, was impaired in wanderers more frequently than nonwanderers.

Unfamiliar environments have been found to increase spatial disorientation. Liu et al. (1991) investigated the spatial orientation skills of 15 older people with Alzheimer's dementia, comparing them to 15 healthy older persons using tests of basic spatial skills, higher cognitive spatial skills, and functional spatial orientation. One basic spatial skill test, right/left orientation, did not differ between elders with dementia and the healthy people, contrary to the previous study.

In the same study by Liu, functional spatial orientation skills were then assessed by asking subjects to navigate in familiar and new environments. People with and without Alzheimer's disease navigated equally well in a familiar environment. But, in the new or unfamiliar environment, the navigation ability of elders with dementia compared to the well elderly declined by 50%. For people with Alzheimer's disease, environmental change alone affects the ability to return safely to a point of origin.

Spatial disorientation as an excess disability is suggested by the findings of Brouwers, Cox, Martin, Chase, and Fedio (1984). In comparing the performance of 4 individuals with Alzheimer's disease to healthy older volunteers on a road map test, no significant differences emerged. The road map test consisted of presenting a simulated street map of a small town. Individuals were asked to imagine traversing a route by indicating whether they would turn left or right at each of 32 chosen points. Although those individuals with Alzheimer's disease were significantly slower in completing the task, and did not perform as well as the healthy older volunteers, their performance was not significantly different. Therefore, when there is difficulty returning to a point of origin, excess disability should be suspected.

METHOD OF ASSESSMENT

The need to understand the effect of spatial disorientation has ramifications for nursing assesment. The ability to identify body parts is assessed through a test of right/left orientation. The procedure is as follows.

At the simple level, the individual is asked to identify one left and one right body part (for example, their right hand and left foot). At a more complex level, the individual is asked to demonstrate awareness of right/left orientation in combination of body parts. For example, the individual is instructed to touch the right ear with the left hand. Finally, to test for left/right orientation in another person, the older person is asked to touch a right and left body part of the assessor (for example, "touch my left hand," "touch my right hand"). If the individual is able to perform these simple tests correctly, spatial orientation abilities regarding right/left orientation to body parts is preserved.

Assessment of the spatial orientation ability to return to the point of origin is achieved through simple observation. For example, is the individual able to return unassisted to their room? If so, then the person retains this aspect of spatial orientation ability.

NURSING ACTIONS

Ability Enhancing

The following ability enhancing nursing actions can enable spatial orientation abilities:

1. encourage free movement;
2. using right/left verbal cues.

When spatial orientation ability is preserved, the individual is encouraged to move about freely in the environment. Some individuals with cognitive impairment may not spontaneously achieve adequate mobilization, despite the ability to orient themselves in space. Therefore, preservation of muscle function by purposefully providing relevant programs is a critical aspect of care.

In a study comparing range of motion of institutionalized, cognitively and noncognitively impaired older persons with age-matched independent elderly, no difference was found in range of motion between the groups. But, following an exercise program, the improvement gained by the institutionalized groups was less than community-dwelling elders, suggesting some excess disability in muscle function in those older persons living in institutions. Muscle function in elders can be maintained through active intervention. It is important to note that older people with cognitive impairment may require greater involvement of nurses to achieve an improvement in function (Pendergast, Calkins, Fisher, & Vickers, 1987).

A simple intervention by the nurse that can enhance retained ability in right/left orientation to body parts the offering of specific left/right verbal cues during daily living activities. For instance, one of our patients with dementia became bewildered during dressing, but with right/left verbal cues, he was able to dress with much greater ease. While dressing, he was instructed as follows: "Put your right arm in this sleeve of your sweater," "place your left foot in this shoe."

NURSING ACTIONS

Ability Compensating

There are several ability-compensating nursing actions which can be employed when spatial orientation abilities are lost. They are:

1. mapping;
2. adaptive clothing and special devices;
3. backward chaining;
4. orientation to the environment;
5. visual barriers;
6. a wanderer's lounge program;
7. nonverbal cues.

When spatial orientation abilities are lost, the intent of underlying nursing care is to act prosthetically.

Although it is important to continue to encourage free mobility, the individual will require supervision if she is unable to return to a point of origin safely. The individual's pattern of movement, and the degree and amount of supervision that is required of nurses, can be determined by mapping movement behavior. Following Snyder, Rupprecht, Pyrek, Brekhus, and Moss (1978), the technique that is employed involves systematically drawing the individual's pattern of space use. Simply follow the individual with a floor map and trace out their walking pattern. The questions to be answered are: How close, or how far, from the point of origin is the individual? Are there intervals at which the individual is close to the point of origin? Then, outline the degree and amount of supervision the individual requires. For instance, a person who retraces the same route can be expected to pass designated areas at predictable intervals, which can then be monitored. In less predictable circumstances, alternative interventions are necessary. These include the use of identifiable clothing or tracking devices.

Special clothing of a specific color and design can alert people to an individual's need for assistance in returning to a point of origin. This approach needs to be considered carefully, as it labels and may stigmatize the individual. Special monitoring or alerting devices can be less stigmatizing. Sensors installed around exits of homes or facilities are activated when individuals wearing a disc around the ankle or wrist approach an exit. The alarm summons the caregivers who can guide the individual away from the exit. In our facility, we observed that many of our residents who wander began to avoid the exits after experiencing the alarm over a period of time. We speculate that this is a learned behavior triggered by the alarm and by the quick and consistent response of the nurses.

Another study indicates that a procedure called "backward chaining" may assist in overcoming spatial disorientation when there is change in environment (McEvoy & Patterson, 1986). This study examined the benefit of this procedure on 15 elders with dementia recently admitted to a day-care program who had difficulty navigating in the new environment. With backward chaining, the navigational skills of these elders improved 100% after one month, and an additional 25 percent after the remaining three months of the study. The comparison group were 15 elders with psychiatric problems. Initially, there was a great deal of difference in the ability of the two groups to maneuver in the environment, the psychiatrically ill individuals having greater ease. Following implementation of the intervention, the differences were minimal.

McEvoy and Patterson define the procedure of spatial reorientation using backward chaining as follows:

> The subject is taken to within the last stage of the trip to a goal, then allowed to do that part on his own. Once this can be done without prompting, the last two stages are left to the subject, and so on, until he is completing the entire trip without prompting. (p. 476)

Let us assume that we wish to help an individual with cognitive impairment to find her way from her room to the cafeteria. The trip is first broken down into smaller manageable distances. The first part of the trip to be learned is that part closest to the intended destination (for example, from the ground elevator to the cafeteria). At this stage, prompting is provided. Each additional part of the trip is managed by providing assistance, but not prompting. When independence has been achieved in the first part of the trip, prompting is then moved to the second part (for example, the unit elevator to the ground-floor elevator) and assistance is given for the remaining details of the trip. This combination of independence, prompting, and assisting continues until the entire trip can be made independently. At the end of the procedure, the person may be able to leave and return to a point of origin.

Another approach to compensate for lost spatial orientation has been studied by Hanley (1981). Training or orientation to the layout of a unit in an institution was compared to sign posts in assisting five older persons with dementia to find their way. Training included the use of a locational map of the unit combined with negotiating a route around the unit. Several months later, large signs were introduced on the unit at which time two additional people with dementia were evaluated. Greater improvement in finding locations was observed following orientation training than following the introduction of signs. Gains made following unit orientation were maintained over a two-week period after the orientation was discontinued, but were lost when these older persons were reevaluated five months later. With unit orientation repeated at this time, spatial orientation improved. Therefore, it seems to be the ongoing orientation to locations in the environment that is ability-compensating when spatial orientation abilities are absent.

Doors may evoke the appropriate behavior of entering or exiting. Unfortunately, this response may lead the older person with dementia into a hazardous situation such as becoming lost from the home or a facility, or evoking a response of anger through invading another individual's personal space. How can individuals be permitted free ambulation when exiting/entering behavior places them at risk of harm?

This question has been explored in 2 studies evaluating the effectiveness of visual barriers to exiting behaviors. In one study, a variety of grid patterns made from beige masking tape were placed in front of an exit door, and were assessed for their effectiveness in discouraging exiting (Hussian & Brown, 1987). The movements of eight older men with dementia were observed. The vertical and horizontal grid patterns led to a reduction in door contacts, but the horizontal pattern was more effective than the vertical. A significant decline in crossing the grid occurred when the grid pattern contained a larger number of strips.

The use of other visual barriers has been evaluated by Namazi, Rosner, and Calkins (1989). Four male and five female persons with Alzheimer's disease living in an institution were observed regarding their movement behavior in response to (1) grid patterns on the floor, (2) cloth panels placed across the door to hide the doorknob, and (3) simple doorknob covers that concealed the knob. In contrast to the findings of Hussian and Brown, the tape grids were ineffective in preventing exit from the unit. The cloth panel barriers eliminated all exiting. The doorknob coverings were more effective than the grid patterns, but less effective than the cloth panels. The cloth panel barriers placed midway on exit doors were shown to be the most ability-compensating.

When spatial orientation abilities are lost, the provision of activities to engage and purposefully focus the attention of the older person with cognitive impairment can be ability-compensating. Activities provided in a lounge for extended periods have been observed to reduce wandering behavior (McGrowder-Lin & Bhatt, 1988). In this study, the program consisted of exercise, discussion, entertainment, and refreshment offered to eight older persons, considered to be problematic to manage, over the change-of-shift time period. As a result of the lounge program, positive behavioral changes were noted in each group member, and wandering decreased.

Restraints may prevent the older person with cognitive impairment from becoming lost, but may not be ability-compensating. These restraints can produce excess disabilities, such as behavioral and physical changes, including agitation, hostility, incontinence, and immobility. Older persons restrained in an acute care setting reported feelings of anger, fear, resistance, humiliation, demoralization, discomfort, resignation, and denial, even though they sometimes agreed with the reasons for restraint (Strumpf & Evans, 1988). These older persons were not cognitively impaired and were able to describe their feelings. Individuals with cognitive impairment may be unable to verbalize their feelings because of language deficits, but would likely experience the same feelings. The caregiving approaches suggested above are more supportive, and may reduce any reliance on restraints.

Nonverbal cues can be ability-compensating regarding the loss of right/left orientation skills. Gentle touch or gesturing can help draw the person's attention to the relevant part of the body.

Loss of the ability for spatial orientation may not be so devastating for the cognitively impaired individual when an ability-compensating nursing approach is assumed. The rewards may be great for both the caregiver and the person, when the person's experience in basic daily living activities is compensated for regardless of the extent of the disease. The person's ability and continuity in the life experience is preserved, and caregiving may not be perceived as quite so burdensome.

• PURPOSEFUL MOVEMENTS •

CLINICAL FEATURES AND THREATENED ABILITIES

Often, individuals with dementia indicate a desire to participate in their care, but are unable to do so. When you ask the older person to pick up the washcloth, she may respond with "okay" but proceed no further. Wells (1979) points this out in his description of the difference between individuals suffering from dementia and other disorders such as depression, which appear as dementia but are not. He characterizes individuals with dementia as struggling to perform tasks, whereas elders with pseudodementia make little effort to perform simple tasks. The ability to undertake purposeful movements may be affected by three clinical features of dementia: ideomotor apraxia, ideational apraxia, and perseveration.

Individuals with ideomotor apraxia have difficulty with movement to command and imitation (Pryse-Phillips & Murray, 1986).

Thus, we may see a willingness to engage in an activity, but also an inability to proceed. If we are not aware of this clinical feature, we may be inclined to interpret the behavior as either a lack of understanding of language or a lack of cooperation, when in fact neither interpretation is accurate. In the instance of the older person's absence of follow-through in picking up the washcloth, she understands the request, but the body is unable to follow the mind.

Ideomotor apraxia was found to be present in individuals with dementia in a study by Della Sala, Lucchelli, and Spinnler (1987). One-third of 18 older persons with mild dementia were found to have ideomotor apraxia in this study. When these individuals were reassessed seven months later, ideomotor apraxia was present in two more people. Compared with other cognitive measures, such as orientation, the authors note that the speed of deterioration of ideomotor apraxia appears to be slow.

Rapcsak, Croswell, and Rubens (1989) evaluated 28 older persons with Alzheimer's dementia on four types of movements and compared their responses to 23 neurologically intact right-handed subjects with respect to the presence of ideomotor apraxia. The four movements included: (1) buccofaccial, such as the ability to stick out the tongue, (2) limb intransitive movements, such as waving good bye or saluting; (3) limb transitive movements, such as using a comb or flipping a coin; and (4) axial movements such as standing up or taking two steps forward. Verbal commands were given initially. Then participants were asked to imitate the examiner, pantomiming these movements. On all four kinds of movements, and for both kinds of instructions, those with Alzheimer's disease performed significantly worse than those in the control group.

Ideational apraxia affects the ability to correctly sequence activities. Pryse-Phillips and Murray (1986) explain ideational apraxia as follows: The individual is aware of what is to be done, but cannot synthesize the movements required to do it, even though she is able to perform the various parts of the whole movement in isolation. They provide an example: Instead of cleaning the pipe, putting tobacco in, lighting it and smoking it, the individual lights the pipe, puts tobacco in it, and then cleans it. Difficulty with serial actions has been found in individuals with Alzheimer's dementia when compared to healthy controls (Rapcsak, Croswell & Rubens, 1989).

Perseveration interferes with stopping and/or completing an activity. Pryse-Phillips and Murray (1986) define perseveration as the continuation or repetition of an activity without the appropriate stimulus, so that the activity persists after the person has consciously attempted to change it. The ability to stop an activity and change to another activity can be affected by dementia. Frontal lobe dysfunction has been implicated in perseveration (Freedman, 1990; Kopelman, 1991).

Shindler, Caplan, and Hier (1984) found only 9 percent of 81 subjects with organic brain disease in their study demonstrated perseveration on verbal activities. Perseveration was not present in healthy control subjects, nor was its presence in the ill subjects related to the severity of the illness. Bayles, Tomoeda, and Kaszniak (1985), on the other hand, found demented patients to verbally perseverate significantly more frequently than normal persons, and the severity of dementia was related to increased perseverations, the latter being a finding of Vitaliano et al. (1984) as well.

Regardless of its frequency, perseveration is important to nurses because its presence has serious implications for caregiving. We have observed both verbal and motor perseveration in our clinical practice. One instance involved an individual with dementia who was noted to run the razor through his hair instead of switching to the use of the comb upon completing shaving. Individuals who perseverate on either verbal or motor activities require assistance to be able to stop one activity and change to another.

In the presence of apraxia and perseveration, the individual's abilities for making purposeful movements are threatened. Specifically, these abilities are: the ability to initiate and follow through on an activity, the ability to persist and appropriately sequence an activity, and the ability to stop and change activities. Methods of assessing for each of these abilities are described below.

Method of Assessment

There are four steps in the assessment of initiation and follow-through abilities. First, the individual is asked to pretend to use an object such as a comb. If the individual has difficulty with the first step, the object is then held in view as a visual cue and the original request is repeated. If the elder is still not able to carry out the instruction, the use of the object is demonstrated by the assessor and the original request is repeated. The ability of the person to complete the command in any of these conditions indicates the presence of initiation and follow-through activities.

The ability to correctly sequence activities of daily living is assessed through direct observation of a simple and a more complex activity. The person is requested to perform a simple activity, such as combing the hair, and a more complex activity, such as putting on socks and shoes. Observe (1) if all component parts of the activity are undertaken in correct sequence, and (2) if the person persists in the activity until it is appropriately completed. Persistence is defined as the attempt to carry to completion activities that are within the person's physical capacity (Clough & Derdiarian, 1980).

Observation of the above purposeful movements also permits assessment of the ability to stop one activity and move to another. For example, can the person stop brushing the teeth and begin handwashing, or does she run the toothbrush across the hands? The former action indicates the ability to stop an activity and move on, while the latter action indicates that this ability has been lost.

Nursing Actions

Ability Enhancing

When the abilities to initiate and follow through, to sequence self-care activities, and to change from one activity to another are present, nursing activities focus on maintaining these abilities. To be enabling, or ability-enhancing:

1. provide the appropriate objects for basic self-care, such as a toothbrush, face cloth and towel, and clothing for dressing;
2. use verbal guidance to support self-care; for example, say "Now that you have completed cleaning your teeth, you may wish to proceed wth bathing";
3. use demonstration as necessary by modelling an activity, such as hair combing.

NURSING ACTIONS

Ability Compensating

When purposeful movement abilities are lost, ability-compensating nursing actions involve:

1. object cueing;
2. touch;
3. direct physical assistance with activities;
4. verbal prompting.

When there is a loss of the ability to initiate and follow through on an activity, it is ability-compensating to directly place the object of importance, such as the toothbrush, in the person's hand. This ability-compensating action serves to cue motor function and may enable the person to proceed independently in cleaning her teeth.

When there is a loss of the ability to persist in or complete basic self-care activities, the nurse or other caregiver can facilitate proper sequencing by the use of gentle touch. Eaton, Mitchell-Bonair, and Friedman, (1986) have demonstrated the effectiveness of touch in their study of the nutritional intake of 21 chronic organic brain syndrome (COBS) patients. In the study, gentle stroking of the forearm was added to verbal encouragement during mealtime. This resulted in a significant increase in the nutritional intake of these elders when compared with another 21 elders with COBS who received verbal encouragement only. Persistence in the activity was facilitated in this simple manner, thereby enabling and preserving the older person's independence in a normal living activity. If cueing and/or the additional intervention of touch does not help, the nurse may need to physically assist with initiating and completing basic living activities.

When the abilities to properly sequence activities, and to stop one activity and move to another activity, have been lost, it is necessary to directly help the individual with sequencing, and to end one activity and transfer to a new activity. Using repeated verbal prompting can be ability compensating. Rinke, Williams, Lloyd, and Smith-Scott (1978) found that prompting or instructions and reinforcements, used separately or in combination, promoted the self-care of elderly, cognitively impaired, nursing home residents in various activities associated with bathing and dressing.

• CONCLUSION •

In this chapter, we have shown some of the ways in which Alzheimer's disease interferes with basic living activities. We have outlined systematic ways of assessing for retained or lost self-care abilities, and have offered suggestions regarding enabling nursing actions. Our premise is that even though an individual's self-care abilities may be threatened or diminished with dementia, enablement as a perspective underlying caregiving can support continued participation of the older person with cognitive impairment in these basic living functions. Another value of this approach is that assistance is provided only when a discrete ability has been identified as lost. Therefore, the whole activity need not be assumed by the caregiver. Excess disability on any of these self-care dimensions can be prevented, and caregiver burden diminished while continuity in life experience and quality of life can be maintained.

• REFERENCES •

Bakchine, S., Lacomblez, L., Palisson, E., Laurent, M., & Derouesne, C. (1989). Relationship between primitive reflexes, extra-pyramidal signs, reflective apraxia and severity of cognitive impairment in dementia of the Alzheimer type. *Acta Neurological Scandinavica, 79,* 38–46.

Barton, E. M., Baltes, M. M., & Orzech, M. J. (1980). Etiology of dependency in older nursing home residents during morning care: The role of staff behavior. *Journal of Personality and Social Psychology, 38*(3), 423–430.

Bayles, K. A., Tomoeda, C. K., & Kaszniak, A. W. (1985). Verbal perseveration of dementia patients. *Brain and Language, 25,* 102–116.

Beck, C. (1988). Measurement of dressing performance in persons with dementia. *The American Journal of Alzheimer's Care and Related Disorders and Research,* 21–25.

Briggs, R. S. J. (1989). Alzheimer's disease: The clinical context. In D. D. Davies (Ed.), *Alzheimer's disease: Toward an understanding of the aetiology and pathogenesis* (pp. 1–8). London: John Libby.

Brouwers, P., Cox, C. , Martin, A., Chase, T., & Fedio, P. (1984). Differential perceptual—spatial impairment in Huntington's and Alzheimer's dementias. *Archives of Neurology, 4,* 1073–1076.

Clough, D. H., & Derdiarian, A. (1980). A behavioral checklist to measure dependence and independence. *Nursing Research, 29*(1), 55–58.

Crystal, H. A., Horoupian, D. S., Katzman, R., & Jotkowitz, S. (1981). Biopsy-proved Alzheimer disease presenting as a right parietal lobe syndrome. *Annals of Neurology, 12*(2): 186–188.

DeLeon, M. J., Potegal, M., & Gurland, B. (1984). Wandering and parietal signs in senile dementia of Alzheimer's type. *Neuropsychobiology, 11,* 155–157.

Della Sala, S., Lucchelli, F., & Spinnler, H. (1987). Ideomotor apraxia in patients with dementia of the Alzheimer type. *Neurology, 234,* 91–93.

Eaton, M., Mitchell-Bonair, I. L., & Friedman, E. (1986). The effect of touch on nutritional intake of chronic organic brain syndrome patients. *Journal of Gerontology, 41*(5), 611–616.

Freeman, M. (1990). Object alternation and orbitofrontal system dysfunction in Alzheimer's and Parkinson's disease. *Brain and Cognition, 14,* 134–143.

Hanley, I. G. (1981). The use of signposts and active training to modify ward disorientation in elderly patients. *Journal of Behavioral Therapy & Experimental Psychiatry, 12*(3), 241–247.

Haxby, J. V., Grady, C. L., Koss, E., Horwitz, B., Schapiro, M., Friedland, R. P., & Rapoport, S. I. (1988). Heterogeneous anterior-posterior metabolic patterns in dementia of the Alzheimer type. *Neurology, 38* (December), 1853–1863.

Hussian, R. (1981). *Geriatric psychology: A behavioral perspective.* New York: Van Nostrand Reinhold.

Hussian, R. A., & Brown, D. C. (1987). Use of two-dimensional grid patterns to limit hazardous ambulation in demented patients. *Journal of Gerontology, 42*(5), 558–560.

Katz, S., Ford, A. B., Moskowitz, R. W., Jackson, B. A., & Jaffe, M. W. (1963). The

Index of ADL: A standardized measure of biological and psychosocial function. *Journal of the American Medical Association, 185,* 914–919.

Koller, W. C., Glatt, S., Wilson, R. S., & Fox, J. H. (1982). Primitive reflexes and cognitive function in the elderly. *Annals of Neurology, 12*(3), 302–304.

Kopelman, M. D. (1991). Frontal dysfunction and memory deficits in the alcoholic Korsakoff syndrome and Alzheimer-type dementia. *Brain, 114,* 117–137.

Kuriansky, J., & Gurland, B. (1976). The performance test of activities of daily living. *International Journal of Aging and Human Development, 1,* 343–352.

Liu, L., Gauthier, L. L, & Gauthier, S. (1991). Spatial disorientation in persons with early senile dementia of the Alzheimer type. *The American Journal of Occupational Therapy, 45*(1), 67–74.

MacLennan, W. J., Ballinger, B. R., McHarg, A., & Oston, S. A. (1987). Dementia and immobility. *Age and Aging, 16,* 1–9.

McEvoy, C. L., & Patterson, R. L. (1986). Behavioral treatment of deficit skills in dementia patients. *The Gerontologist, 26*(5), 475–478.

McGrowder-Lin, R., & Bhatt, A. (1988). A wanderer's lounge program for nursing home residents with Alzheimer's disease. *The Gerontologist, 28*(5), 607–609.

Mahoney, F. I., & Barthel, D. W. (1965). Functional evaluation: the Barthel index. *Maryland State Medical Journal, 14,* 61–65.

Miller, C. A. (1990). *Nursing care of older adults: Theory and practice.* Glenview, IL: Scott, Foresman/Little, Brown.

Namazi, K. H., Rosner, T. T., & Calkins, M. P. (1989). Visual barriers to prevent ambulatory Alzheimer's patients from exiting through an emergency door. *The Gerontologist, 29*(5), 699–702.

Pendergast, D. R., Calkins, E. E., Fisher, N. M., and Vickers, R. (1987). Muscle rehabilitation in nursing home residents with cognitive impairment: A pilot study. *The American Journal of Alzheimer's Care and Related Disorders and Research, 2,* 20–25.

Pryse-Phillips, W., & Murray, T. J. (1986). *Essential neurology* (3rd ed.). New York: Medical Examination Publishing Company.

Rapcsak, S. Z., Croswell, S. C., & Rubens, A. B. (1989). Apraxia in Alzheimer's disease. *Neurology, 39,* 664–668.

Reed, B. R., Jagust, W. J. & Seab, J. P. (1989). Mental status as a predictor of daily function in progressive dementia. *The Gerontologist, 29,* 804–807.

Rinke, C. L., Williams, J. J., Lloyd, K. E., & Smith-Scott, W. (1978). The effects of prompting and reinforcement on self-bathing by elderly residents of a nursing home. *Behavior Therapy, 9,* 873–881.

Shindler, A. G., Caplan, L. R., & Hier, D. B. (1984). Intrusions and reservations. *Brain and Language, 23,* 148-158.

Snyder, L. H., Rupprecht, P., Pyrek, J., Brekhus, S. & Moss, T. (1978). Wandering. *The Gerontologist, 18*(3), 272–280.

Strumpf, N. E., & Evans, L. K. (1988). Physical restraint of the hospitalized elderly: Perceptions of patients and nurses. *Nursing Research, 37*(3), 132–137.

Tweedy, J., Reding, M., Garcia, C., Schulman, P., Deutsch, G., & Antin, S. (1982). Significance of cortical disinhibition signs. *Neurology, 32,* 169–173.

Villeneuve, A., Turcotte, J., Bouchard, M., Cote, J. M., & Jus, A. (1974, January 19).

Release phenomena and iterative activities in psychiatric geriatric patients. *CMA Journal,* p 110.

Vitaliano, P. P., Breen, A. R., Russo, J., Albert, M., Vitiello, M., & Prinz, P. N. (1984). The clinical utility of the dementia rating scale for assessing Alzheimer patients. *Journal of Chronic Disorders, 17*(9/10), 743–753.

Weaverdyck, S. E. (1987). A cognitive intervention protocol for dementia: Its derivation from and application to a neuro-psychological case study of Alzheimer's disease. *Dissertation Abstracts International, 48,* 576-B.

Wells, C. D. (1979). Pseudodementia. *American Journal of Psychiatry, 136,* 895.

THREE

SOCIAL ABILITIES

S OCIABILITY IS AT THE CORE OF HUMAN EXISTENCE. SOCIABIL-
ity refers to "the quality or state of being sociable"; to be
sociable means "inclined by nature to companionship with others of
the same species" (Webster's Ninth New Collegiate Dictionary,
1987). This definition implies that older persons with dementia
continue to be social beings, as they have lived a lifetime in a social
world. There are many ways, however, in which dementia may
shatter the person's sociability, as perceptions of self, of others, and
of the world are altered by the disease. Consequently, the social
integrity and humanness of the individual may be threatened.

We believe that careful attention to the social abilities of the
individual with cognitive impairment can assist with continued
sociability if we understand how dementia affects these abilities.
For older persons with dementia who live in institutions, it is
important to also consider how institutional factors interfere with
established sociability patterns. Because Goffman's (1961) identifi-

cation of the characteristics of institutions, attention has been given to humanizing routines, policies, and interactions between caregivers and those receiving care in long-term care facilities. These concepts are critical to the care of individuals with dementia, and more progress is still needed for the true individualization of care and the preservation of sociability.

We define "social abilities" as those capacities used to interact with others and to engage in various activities using socially prescribed behaviors. The abilities that we discuss in this chapter are those required to engage in or respond to social cues, and to behave normatively in social contexts. "Social cues" refers to familiar, everyday exchanges made by individuals to acknowledge one another. "Social contexts" are the situations, events, and activities that are associated with interactions among individuals. Behavioral disturbances and lowered stress threshold that may accompany dementia are discussed as factors impinging on sociability. Incorporating cues into nursing practice and creating appropriate contexts can enhance the social abilities of the older person with dementia, and offset dysfunctional behavior or a lowered tolerance to stress. Moreover, we assume that by enhancing or compensating for the abilities of individuals with cognitive impairment, we can prevent or reverse excess disability, particularly, social isolation.

• SOCIAL CUES •

CLINICAL FEATURES AND THREATENED ABILITIES

Social cues are culturally ingrained behavioral repertoires that we engage in when meeting or acknowledging another person. In North America, for example, when meeting or addressing someone we don't know, the behavioral repertoire includes verbal cues, such as "Hello, Mrs. Brown, my name is Joan Smith," to which the familiar and anticipated response might be "Hello, Joan, I'm pleased to meet you. Please call me Mary." Nonverbal cues such as eye contact, smiling, and extending a handshake might be included in this ritualistic behavior pattern. In this example, if Joan Smith had not included the "Hello" or the smile, the behavior would have given a different message, causing Mrs. Brown to be less forthcoming in her response. Perhaps a more formal response would have been offered, or she would have been less willing to further engage in conversation. Similarly, if Mrs. Brown had not extended a handshake, or had merely responded with an unsmiling "hello," Joan Smith would not have pursued further conversation and might have hastily retreated from Mrs. Brown. Social cues are subtle, conventional behaviors that we use to initiate our social interactions with others. Because they are culturally embodied, any deviations in response give powerful messages.

For social interactions to proceed, individuals must be able to attend to social cues. This ability, however, is threatened with dementia. Attention-giving deficits is the clinical feature of interest with respect to the ability to use social cues. Attention deficits have been found in older persons with Alzheimer's disease (Huff et al., 1987), and have the potential to disable the individual's participation in social interactions. "Distracted," "noncompliant," or "unresponsive" are terms that may be applied to individuals with cognitive impairment who have difficulty with giving attention. In order for nurses to be prosthetic and support the social abilities of persons with cognitive impairment, a further understanding of the effect of Alzheimer's disease on attention is imperative to avoid unnecessary labelling.

The components of attention as described by Posner and Boies (1971) include: (1) alertness, (2) the ability to select information from one source rather than another, and (3) a central processing capacity. To give attention requires a responsiveness to external stimuli such as people, activities or objects; receptivity to particular stimuli, while blocking input from concurrent but contextually unrelated stimuli; and demonstrating behaviors in relation to a stimulus. For attention-giving to occur in social situations, individuals must have an awareness of another person, decide to sustain a focus on the other to the exclusion of simultaneous happenings in the environment, and acknowledge the other person.

Contrary to Huff et al.'s (1987) findings, the ability to receive attention and to discriminate with respect to the quality of a stimulus has been shown to be preserved in individuals with cognitive impairment (Hoffman, Platt, Barry, & Hamill, 1985). Hoffman, Platt, Barry, and Hamill evaluated the responses of 54 older persons to unpleasant and pleasant stimuli: 10 without dementia, 7 with mild dementia, and 37 with severe dementia. The pleasant stimulation consisted of: (1) a visual component, where the examiner was relaxed, smiling, and had an open facial expression; (2) an auditory stimulation, where the examiner spoke the subject's name in a soft, pleasant tone; and (3) a tactile component, consisting of touch and clasping the subject's hand warmly in a handshake. The unpleasant stimulation was conveyed as follows. Visually, the investigator frowned and had an angry facial expression. The subject's name was then spoken in a harsh, abrupt manner, creating an unpleasant auditory stimulus. Unpleasant touch was conveyed by grasping the subject's wrist firmly. To determine the responses of these older individuals to the pleasant and unpleasant stimuli, changes in their posture, head orientation, head adjustment, facial expression, and eye contact were recorded. The specific interest was in the older person's focus of movement and attention in the direction of the examiner or away from the examiner. Positive scores were given for movement toward, and negative scores were given for movement away.

The researchers found that there were no differences between the responses of older persons with severe, mild, or no cognitive impairment, suggesting that dementia may have no impact on the way in which an older person responds to unpleasant or pleasant stimulation. For all subjects, the response to the pleasant stimulus was found to be one of friendliness and approachability, conveyed by head and body movement toward the examiner, eye contact, and smiling or relaxing of the facial muscles. For the unpleasant stimulus, all subjects reacted with an unfriendly withdrawal response.

Behaviors such as moving the head and body away from the examiner, closing eyes or looking elsewhere, and wrinkling of the head and frowning were indicative of this response. Even older persons with severe dementia were found to be sensitive to the emotional undertones in the environment. From this study we learn that older persons with cognitive impairment are able to give and receive attention conducive to sociability, and that even those who are severely impaired are sensitive to the social environment; hence, this environment should be as pleasant as possible to facilitate social interaction.

The limited research on attention-giving behaviors is equivocal with respect to the occurrence of attention deficits in dementia. Regardless, it is important to consider the ability to give and receive attention in the assessment of social abilities, as this ability is basic to engaging in social cues and to preserving sociability.

Method of Assessment

We assess for the social ability to give and receive attention by providing familiar, everyday, social salutations. First, the individual is greeted with "hello" or "good morning." Her response may be: (1) a verbal reply, (2) a smile only, (3) eye contact only, (4) muttering, or (5) no change in behavior. Next, the individual's response to another familiar social greeting, "How are you?" is assessed. Responses that are recorded are: (1) a verbal reply, (2) a verbal reply which is unclear, (3) a nonverbal response, such as an eye gaze, a nod, or a smile, or (4) no change in behavior.

The social cues of a personal introduction and a handshake are also included in the assessment of the individual's abilities to give and to receive attention. In the assessment, the nurse introduces herself by name and observes for the following behaviors: (1) name repetition or self-introduction, that is, the individual repeats the nurse's name or gives her own name, (2) there is a facial response; the individual either nods, smiles, or looks, (3) there is a body language response; the individual leans forward, (4) the person mumbles, or (5) there is no response. With the social cue of a handshake, the nurse offers her hand to the individual and observes for the following: (1) the individual grasps the offered hand (self-initiated), (2) the person requires the nurse to initiate or take the hand (other-initiated), (3) the individual initiates letting go, or (4) there is no response.

The social cues of greetings, inquiry, introduction, and handshaking are behaviors that nurses use all the time to initiate interaction. When using these cues for assessment purposes, it is necessary to slow down and offer each social cue in sequence with pauses between them to allow the person time to respond. Reaction time in older persons with Alzheimer's disease, even to a single stimulus, has been reported as slower than in healthy older persons (Pirozzolo, Christensen, Ogle, Hansch, & Thompson, 1981). Adequate time is required, as well, to permit the nurse to observe and record the response accurately.

NURSING ACTIONS

Ability Enhancing

When older persons with cognitive impairment retain the ability to give and receive attention indicated by any of the assessment findings, except when the individual fails to respond, the following ability-enhancing nursing actions can preserve and increase these abilities:

1. the use of a conventional greeting on each contact;
2. the planning of frequent one-to-one interactions;
3. involvement in group activities;
4. the inclusion of animals in the social environment.

Because of the reduction of recent memory with Alzheimer's disease (Clark 1980), the frequency with which nurses use a conventional greeting on contact is unimportant. A greeting can be repeated over and over again, and each time that it is offered, it can elicit or enhance the ability of the person to initiate or respond to greetings. We know of one elderly woman with very advanced Alzheimer's disease who had not responded verbally for a prolonged period of time. After a week of her nurse using a conventional greeting many times a day, the woman began to respond with verbal greetings herself. This simple behavior significantly influenced both the number and frequency of social interactions she then had with other nurses. We speculate that the increase in social interaction with others provided comfort or solace to this person in her otherwise silent and isolated world. Familiar social cues can also enable the nurse to gain the elder's attention in day-to-day caregiving activities.

When the older person is attentive to social salutations, the ability to engage in one-to-one interaction may be present. If so, it is important to plan frequent one-to-one interactions. It is valuable to accompany each greeting with a smile, conveying a pleasant message to the person with whom we intend to interact (Hoffman et al., 1985). Use the person's name and introduce yourself with each contact, keeping in mind the decline in recent memory. Because of the enhancing effects of touch, we also initiate each contact with a handshake, a highly familiar social cue.

Close proximity in visiting situations, that is, a one-to-one visiting situation, has been found to increase the social behaviors of smiling and talking (Hendy, 1987). Families and others might be informed of the value of one-on-one visits for individuals with cognitive impairment.

When individuals are responsive and comfortable in one-to-one interaction, assess their ability to participate in group activities. Witte (1987) reports that nine older persons with cognitive impairment involved in a cognitive-linguistic program were able to be attentive for 30–45 minutes.

Animals in the environment may also enhance attending behaviors. Kongable, Buckwalter, and Stolley (1989) reported an increase in smiles, laughter, and the attending behaviors of looking, leaning, touching, verbalizations, and name-calling in 10 older men and 2 older women with Alzheimer's disease, when a dog was brought into the environment. These changes were observed both when the dog visited weekly and when it become a permanent resident on the unit. These investigators concluded that companion animals may serve as a social behavior catalyst. Along with individual and group activities, animals can maintain and improve the ability of older persons with cognitive impairment to engage in or respond to social cues.

Francis and Baly (1986) report an improvement not only in social behavior, but also in the psychological well-being of individuals with and without Alzheimer's disease when plush animals were introduced into a nursing home environment. This suggests that inanimate as well as animate objects can enhance sociability and well-being, provided that individuals are not placed at risk of infantilization.

Nursing Actions

Ability Compensating

Nursing actions that are compensating for persons with cognitive impairment when the abilities of giving and receiving attention are lost are similar to the ability-enhancing nursing actions suggested above, and include:

1. attending behaviors;
2. touch.

Because it has been shown that individuals with severe dementia are responsive to pleasant and unpleasant greetings (Hoffman et al., 1985), we assume that the ability to give and receive attention is dormant, rather than lost, even though social responsiveness may not be immediately apparent.

Support for this assumption is provided by Rosendahl and Ross (1982). They questioned the influence of attending behaviors on the ability of older persons to respond to a mental status questionnaire. Two groups of 25 elders who resided in a chronic care facility were assessed for their response to a mental status questionnaire. One group received attending behaviors and the other did not. Attending behaviors were those that communicated attention or interest in another person, and included initiating and maintaining good eye contact, practicing physical relaxation, maintaining comfortable posture and natural movements, and using comments that followed directly upon topics the client had introduced. Persons who received attending behaviors in conjunction with the mental status questionnaire scored significantly higher than those who did not receive the attending behaviors. These same authors replicated these findings with a different sample of 50 older persons. Their studies imply that attending behaviors can enable elders to focus and sustain attention on a stimulus.

The use of touch has been found to be compensating for those who have lost the ability to focus or give attention. Two nurses, Langland and Panicucci (1982), studied the response to requests of older people with cognitive impairment. For one half of these elders, the request was combined with light touch on the forearm. With the remaining half, the request was given verbally only. These nurses were interested in seeing whether touch had an effect on the giving of attention. This effect was measured by: (1) facial expression (including smiling, nodding the head up and down, raising the eyebrows, or blinking the eyes); (2) eye contact, that is, the subject looked toward the nurse; and (3) body movement, including touching the nurse or turning the body toward her. Thirty-two elderly women residing in an intermediate nursing care facility participated in this study. The women with cognitive impairment who received touch responded with more attending behaviors. Touch was an approach that was compensating for these subjects, and is considered in practice as an ability-compensating nursing approach for older persons with cognitive impairment.

• SOCIAL CONTEXTS •

Social contexts are situations associated with the sociability of individuals. These include simple one-to-one conversations that might involve humor, formal and informal group activities, the attending of social events, such as concerts, or simply listening to music. An individual's inclination to participate socially with others in these contexts may be affected by dementia. With cognitive impairment, sociability can be affected by numerous clinical features of the disease. Some of these are discussed in relation to interactional and interpretive abilities. In this chapter, the specific clinical features examined in relation to sociability are impaired conversation and confabulation, and the potential inability to appreciate humor and music. The social abilities affected by these clinical features of the disease are conversational abilities and the abilities to appreciate humor and music, all of which represent social contexts for maintaining sociability. General behavioral disturbances and a progressively lowered stress threshold (Hall & Buckwalter, 1987), both thought to occur with Alzheimer's disease, are discussed at the end of the chapter as additional threats to social abilities.

CONVERSATIONAL ABILITIES

CLINICAL FEATURES AND THREATENED ABILITIES

Impairment of conversational abilities with dementia affects the individual's ability to interact using socially prescribed behaviors. Engaging in social exchanges or conversation involves the use of the rules of language, of which utterances, turns, topics, and the cooperation principle are examples (Hutchinson & Jensen, 1980). Utterances are separate linguistic units, one word or a series of words, with pauses or terminal intonations. A turn is one or more consecutive utterances by the speaker. A person in conversation will participate or take a turn after another person finishes speaking. A series of utterances by one or more speakers relating to the same general theme constitutes a topic. When participants make appropriate contributions to discourse, at the appropriate time, and according to the accepted purpose or direction of the conversation, they are upholding the cooperation principle. In the presence of cognitive impairment, some of these skills become impoverished, and hence the ability to converse in a socially acceptable fashion is diminished.

The conversational behavior of five elderly female patients who had symptoms of dementia was compared to that of five elderly female patients who had normal intellectual functioning (Hutchinson & Jensen, 1980). In analyzing conversations between each subject and an examiner, it was found that the number of utterances during 45 minutes of conversation was less for the people with dementia than for those without. A similar finding was reported in the comparison of six older individuals with Alzheimer's disease with six older persons in good health (Ripich & Terrell, 1988). Regarding turn taking, Hutchinson and Jensen found that women with dementia initiated more turns in the conversation than those without. The appearance of fewer utterances per turn by those with dementia suggests that their ability to elaborate on various topics is reduced. Although the amount of information on any given topic may be less, the ability to converse is not necessarily diminished. Ripich and Terrell's study illustrated that the women who had dementia did not differ significantly from the healthy women with respect to the continuation of the topic of conversation. Thus, although the give and take involved in communication may not be affected by the presence of cognitive impairment, the content itself may be influenced. This may affect the opportunities that elders with dementia have to converse. Cognitively normal individuals may be less likely to converse with someone whose conversational content is lacking. This puts elders with cognitive impairment at risk for the excess disability of social isolation.

The other clinical feature of dementia that may influence the conversational abilities of older persons is confabulation. Confabulation is defined as the telling of improbable stories (Joslyn, Grundvig, & Chamberlain, 1978). When confabulation is present, the person may relate activities or events in their conversations which in all probability did not occur in the recent past. When given drawings, individuals who confabulate provide a great deal more detail than those who do not.

In Jocelyn et al.'s study of confabulation, 16 older people with chronic brain syndrome were compared with 16 people diagnosed with schizophrenia. Confabulation was measured by the number of embellishments or additional features made on drawings taken from the Memory for Design Test. The confabulators in each group differed from the nonconfabulators in that they embellished the drawings almost twice as frequently. The adding of detail has been observed in practice in verbal conversation. Although the content of conversation may be of dubious accuracy for individuals with cognitive impairment, the detailed content can act as a basis for continued conversation, thus preserving sociability.

METHOD OF ASSESSMENT

To assess the individual's response to conversation, a topic is initiated by the nurse based on the individual's past or current interests. The person's response is recorded in relation to: (1) the topic; stays on topic, relates improbable events, or is unresponsive, (2) verbal behavior; makes distinct verbal responses, indistinct verbal responses, or no verbal response, (3) nonverbal behavior; takes turns, looks, listens or nods, is unresponsive, or moves away from the nurse. Conversational abilities are considered present except when there is no response.

NURSING ACTIONS

Ability Enhancing

When conversational abilities are present:

1. the development of rapport, and
2. the use of purposeful conversation are undertaken to preserve these abilities.

These two nursing approaches afford a supportive social context, and are assistive in maintaining sociability.

Rapport was found to be an effective means of achieving social interaction in elders with dementia (Porszt-Miron, Florian, & Burton, 1988). Two groups of three older women with cognitive impairment participated in a 4-week program consisting of a variety of activities: light exercise, arts and crafts, cooking, and music. Rapport was developed with one group of these women by the group leaders, who used attending behaviors as used by Rosendahl and Ross (1982). The other group of women did not receive attending behaviors. Assessments of both groups were conducted weekly by the group leaders for 3 weeks before and after the intervention in the experimental group. A pattern of increased consistency in appropriate verbal responses was reported for those persons with whom rapport had been established. An additional benefit of the program was the decline in inappropriate physical behaviors. Rapport can be seen, then, as having an enabling effect on social interaction, and hence may help to maintain sociability. Rapport, however, is dependent upon consistency in nurses.

Purposeful conversation can preserve sociability for older persons with cognitive impairment. Conversational skills and group participation have been reported to be enhanced by a cognitive-linguistic program focusing on dialogue in a group of eight women with Alzheimer's disease (Witte, 1987). During a subsequent period of 1½ years, these women demonstrated continued abilities in generating phrases and sentences relevant to the topic of conversation. They also continued to be active in initiation of conversational turns.

In our view, participation in conversation takes precedence over the content of conversation. When the conversation of the person with cognitive impairment is confabulatory, we continue to promote conversational abilities and to look for themes in the content, which we can then explore with the person.

NURSING ACTIONS

Ability Compensating

When conversational abilities are absent or possibly dormant, ability-compensating nursing approaches involve the use of *resocialization groups.*

Resocialization groups have been found to be ability-compensating in that they provide a safe social context, in which the amount and kind of stimulation can be regulated and dormant social abilities can be reactivated. With these goals in mind, two nurses provided resocialization groups to determine if changes in verbal interaction resulted (Gray & Stevenson, 1980). They worked with 17 persons with cognitive impairment who were divided into three groups. The first was ambulatory and aware of social norms. The second group was nonambulatory and aware of social norms. The third group was nonambulatory and unaware of social norms; these persons were described as being loud and fighting over each other's food. The three groups separately received a resocialization program that included a welcome and introduction, orientation to date, time and place without pressure to learn, refreshments served by group members, discussion based on pictures of the food served and other topics, and closure. They met once a week for a period of 45–50 minutes over a 4-month period; caregivers acted as group leaders, and volunteers as back-up. After 4 months, it was found that there were changes in the verbal responses within each group. The number of verbal responses increased in all groups. An increase in the number of interactions between members of the group was also recorded, especially in the third group, who were neither ambulatory nor aware of social norms. These findings raise an interesting question: Were the shouting, fighting, and other inappropriate verbal behaviors of the third group of cognitively impaired persons due to dementia, or were they indicators of excess disability as a result of the disuse of social skills? In using a similar approach daily for 2 weeks with 10 individuals with cognitive impairment, we found improvements both in mental status and physical and behavioral function.

Resocialization is an ability-compensating approach that can possibly reverse excess disability. It offers a prosthetic social context to preserve conversational abilities and prevent social isolation.

HUMOR APPRECIATION

CLINICAL FEATURES AND THREATENED ABILITIES

Little information exists regarding the relationship of humor to the sociability of older persons with cognitive impairment. Humor often draws on the familiar with unexpected twists. An incongruous or unpredictable ending or punch line to a particular train of thought is characteristic of humor. Because humor draws on the cognitive processes of memory, judgment, and relating to the abstract, it can be argued that humor is not appropriate for older persons with dementia. Adasiak (1989), however, provides several anecdotal reports of older persons with Alzheimer's disease who responded positively to humor. It is our belief that humor can create a prosthetic social context and facilitate sociability.

Sullivan and Deane (1988) have reported on 63 humorous incidents occurring in a psychogeriatric setting. Although the kind of patients in this setting were not specifically reported, there is a great likelihood that some of those people were suffering from cognitive impairment. Of 63 humor incidents, 32 were initiated by patients. These were most often joke-telling, sharing of humorous incidents, or plays on words. We have observed the use of play on words by an older person with cognitive impairment in our clinical practice. This occurred in a social group in which people spent time throwing two balls back and forth. On one occasion, one ball bounced off the other ball, and a resident responded by saying "That's what I call being on the ball." Observations such as these have prompted the exploration of the response of persons with cognitive impairment to humor (Dawson, 1992).

In our practice, we assessed 30 older men with cognitive impairment for their response to verbal humor (a joke) and visual humor (a cartoon). Three jokes and four cartoons were selected on the basis of the gender and cohort preference of 10 older men with no cognitive impairment. The men with cognitive impairment were able to respond to both the visual and verbal humor. Responses to the joke were examined in terms of laughter, smiling, or changing facial expression, unexpected reaction, or showing no response. Nineteen of 29 older men with cognitive impairment (64%) responded to the joke either by laughing at the punch line or smiling. An additional interesting observation has been that even though the joke may not have been completely understood, the social context of telling the joke seemed to serve as a cue for these older men to laugh. It also often acted as a stimulus for them to tell a joke or make a humorous comment. The response to the cartoon was similar to that of the joke. Eighteen of 30 older men with cognitive impairment (60%) responded to the cartoon to some extent by laughing out loud, laughing quietly, or smiling. These responses indicate that cognitive impairment does not necessarily preclude the ability to respond to humor. Indeed, using humor can elicit a variety of social behaviors that are reinforcing to the social well-being of elders with cognitive impairment.

METHOD OF ASSESSMENT

Responsiveness to humor is assessed in two ways. One is through a visual stimulus, a cartoon, and the other is by way of a verbal or auditory stimulus, a joke. The cartoon selected by the gentlemen we surveyed is shown in Figure 3.1. The individual's response is observed for: (1) laughing out loud or making relevant comments, (2) laughing quietly, (3) smiling, or (4) no response. The joke used in the assessment of humor is the following:

> A kangaroo walked into a bar and ordered a beer. The bartender said, "That will be $5.00, please." A little later the bartender went to the kangaroo and said, "We don't get many kangaroos in here." The kangaroo replied, "I am not surprised at these prices!"

It is a short joke that is intended to be nonprejudicial and noncontroversial. The nurse maintains a straight face at the punch line, in order that the joke, rather than the nurse's facial expression be the stimulus evoking a response. Laughing, making relevant comments, changing one's facial expression, or making an unexpected response, such as crying at the punch line, reflect responsiveness to the joke. Humor is present for the cartoon when laughing, smiling or comments are observed.

NURSING ACTIONS

Ability Enhancing

The purposeful use of humor may be ability-enhancing in terms of reducing inappropriate social behaviors and maintaining sociability. Although a study by Tennant (1990) did not focus on the cognitively impaired, the findings do indicate that older individuals attending a day center who participated in a humor group experienced a significant decrease in agitation and loneliness. Furthermore, these people reported satisfaction with the humor-group

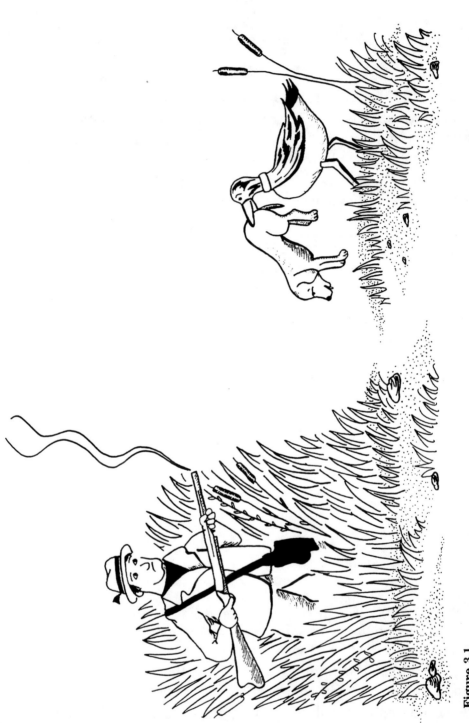

Figure 3.1
This cartoon is intended to assess humor appreciation.

experience. The group preferred a live comedian, and situation comedies, such as "I Love Lucy" and "The Honeymooners," over other forms of humor; this may be related to the use of laugh tracks in these programs. Because older persons with cognitive impairment are reported to be responsive to humor, and because humor, and laughter in particular is believed to have numerous physiological (Peter & Dana, 1982) and communication (Sullivan & Deane, 1988) benefits, humor is employed as an ability-enhancing nursing approach.

Nursing Actions

Ability Compensating

Even when persons with Alzheimer's disease are found to be unresponsive to humor, humor may be used to create a positive social context for social interaction and social well-being. We speculate that the use of more concrete forms of humor, such as a clown's nose and a laughing mirror, might be ways of eliciting humor in persons unresponsive to the joke or cartoon. In view of humor's potential value in ability-enhancing behaviors, it would be valuable to study the responsiveness of cognitively impaired individuals over time to humor, and to the changing nature of social exchanges when humor is present.

MUSIC APPRECIATION

Clinical Features and Threatened Abilities

Music, as well as humor, can be a context that facilitates social interrelationships and personal well-being. Music is considered the most social of the arts, and is thought to be an integrating force that can facilitate communication among disparate groups of people

(Glynn, 1986). Listening to music may create an opportunity to share social experiences among individuals, or it may simply be a personally pleasurable experience. Music has been reported to have beneficial social and physiological effects (Norberg, Melin, & Asplund, 1986). Through a case-study method, these researchers illustrated the powerful impact of music as a stimulus for reaching others or achieving personal well-being. In their study of two elders in the final stages of Alzheimer's disease, music was found to be the only stimulus to which any contact or response could be elicited as measured by heart rate, respirations, eye blinking, and mouth movements.

METHOD OF ASSESSMENT

An individual's response to music is assessed by careful observation of the individual during the playing of tape-recorded music, and in collaboration with the family. Selections of big band, marching, and classical music represent different rhythms and kinds of music that might be appreciated by this older cohort of individuals. Older persons with cognitive impairment are considered to be responsive to music if any of the following behaviors are observed: (1) becomes quiet during music, (2) makes sounds, such as singing, humming, or comments on the music, or (3) moves the body by tapping hands or feet, or swaying. A lack of change in behavior is reflective of unresponsiveness to music.

NURSING ACTIONS

Ability Enhancing

When the ability to appreciate music is retained, ability-enhancing actions offered are:

1. the opportunity to listen to music;
2. group singing activities.

As part of daily living activities, we suggest the incorporation of music of the older person's choice. What little we know of the relationship between music and cognitive impairment suggests that music appreciation persists and can be therapeutic.

Group singing has been reported to be more effective than a discussion group for persons with Alzheimer's disease in increasing social and physical behaviors (Millard & Smith, 1989). Two groups of 5 persons with the disease were compared on physical and social behaviors for 30 minutes following a singing group and a discussion group. Although both group situations resulted in an increased frequency of appropriate physical and social behaviors, the greatest increase was reported for the singing group.

NURSING ACTIONS

Ability Compensating

Ability-compensating nursing approaches when individuals are unresponsive to music may be:

1. the continued use of music in the environment;
2. musical vibration.

What little we know of music appreciation and Alzheimer's disease suggests that even when the older person is found to be unresponsive to music on assessment, it may still be beneficial to include music in the environment. Bergman (1986) cites an anecdote exemplifying the power of music to affect social behavior:

> An aide in a psycho-geriatric unit once asked me to watch a "miracle." She led me to a doubled-over, withdrawn, frail old lady. The aide started singing some Yiddish lullabies. The old lady straightened up in her chair, brushed back her hair, and

burst into song. The aide had discovered this response to song by chance, when she was humming to herself while cleaning the room. Discussion with the family revealed that the patient had been a concert soloist in her home in Poland. This incident generated some additional awareness of the patient, now seen as Mrs. M. (p. 363).

This poignant story shows the compensating nature of music. To be prosthetic, the music selected should be based on a knowledge of the person's music preferences.

The experience of musical vibration can also be ability-compensating (Clair & Bernstein, 1990). The responses of six men with Alzheimer's disease who were observed to be generally unresponsive were compared under three different music conditions. In the first situation, the men played a drum that was placed on their knees. Second, the men played a drum that was placed in front of them. Third, the men engaged in singing along with a music therapist. The music condition that was engaged in over the longest period was drum-playing when the drum was on the knees. The authors concluded that vibrational tactile stimulation may facilitate active music participation. The playing of musical instruments that generate vibrations may thus be another ability-compensating approach.

In summary, opportunities to engage in conversation, humor, and music have the potential to maintain the sociability of elders with cognitive impairment. The ability-enhancing and compensating nursing activities suggested above can potentially contribute to an improved quality of life for these persons, especially those who must live out their lives in long-term care facilities.

BEHAVIORAL DISTURBANCES, COGNITIVE IMPAIRMENT, AND SOCIAL ABILITIES

"My mother often reacts to me with anger since she became ill." "Mr. Jones hit me the other day." These are behaviors of older persons with cognitive impairment that have been described by family and health caregivers. Behavioral disturbances interfere with the sociability of older persons with dementia, and create challenges for them and for their caregivers in daily living.

Many behavioral disturbances have been associated with dementia, including aggression, angry outbursts, hitting or hurting others, and agitation (Alessi, 1991). The prevalence of these and other behavioral disturbances has been reported to be high, as determined from reports of family members and health caregivers (Haley, Brown, & Levine, 1987), and to vary from home to institution and between institutions (Alessi, 1991; Girling & Berrios, 1990).

The behavioral disturbance of aggression, defined as behavior liable to cause physical injury to others, was reported in 20% of 178 older people with dementia (Burns, Jacoby, & Levy, 1990). Similarly, Swearer, Drachman, O'Donnell, and Mitchell (1988) noted that 21% of 126 older persons with dementia demonstrated aggressive behaviors. Eighty-three percent of these individuals showed one or more of the nine troublesome behaviors targeted in their study.

Agitation is another disturbing behavior frequently reported in the literature. In a study by Cohen-Mansfield, Marx, and Rosenthal (1989), 93% of individuals living in a nursing home manifested one or more agitated behaviors at least once a week. Although the diagnoses of these individuals is not reported, it is assumed that a significant number of those studied ($n = 408$) had cognitive impairment, which, as noted in the introduction, is known to affect more than 50 percent of those living in nursing homes. A number of agitation behaviors tended to coexist within individuals, including aggressive behavior such as hitting and kicking, nonaggressive behavior such as pacing, disrobing, and repetitive questions, verbally agitated behavior such as complaining, and hiding or hoarding things.

There is no clear understanding of the etiology or pathology of disturbing behaviors (Swearer, Drachman, O'Donnell, & Mitchell,

1988). Yet some correlations have been made between pathological changes in the brain and behavior, for example, between temporal lobe atrophy and aggression. An increase in behavioral problems has been noted to occur with heightened severity of the disease (Burns, Jacoby, & Levy, 1990; Teri, Larson, & Reifler, 1988). A decrease in appropriate social behaviors has been associated with a rise in the number of drugs consumed (Allen, Yanchick, Cook, & Foss, 1990). Agitation and other disturbing behaviors are thought to be related to increased stress induced by environmental stimuli (Hall & Buckwalter; Lawton & Nahemow, 1973) suggesting the presence of excess disability. Given the current state of knowledge, it is difficult to determine when behavioral disturbances reflect excess disability, which is not part of the disease, or actual disability, arising from the pathology of the disease.

Hall and Buckwalter (1987) hypothesize that behavioral disturbances in elders with dementia may arise as a consequence of the persistent stress of unobtainable mastery secondary to a progressively lowered stress threshold. In their model, the older person's social behavior alters when she experiences the stress of not being able to contend with or master the environment. There is increased psychomotor activity and avoidance behavior. If the stress continues, both dysfunctional or catastrophic behavior, such as wandering, and violent or extremely agitated and anxious behavior occurs. When the environmental stress is alleviated, the older person returns to a state of sociability. In other words, sociability can be maintained when the stress or stimulation in the environment does not exceed the competence of the individual.

We believe that social behavioral disturbances may be mostly excess disability, as preserved social graces in 72%–80% of individuals with Alzheimer's disease has been reported (Girling & Berrios, 1990). In a survey in our own setting, the responses of 15 persons with cognitive impairment and 15 persons without were compared on the Minimum Social Behavior Scale (Dastoor, 1975) which incorporates responses to questions such as "hello" and "how are you." and observations of behaviors such as "drooling without noticing." Seventy percent of those with cognitive impairment were found to have preserved social graces.

It is only after nursing care which is enabling in orientation has been consistently offered and found to be ineffective that behavioral disturbances might be attributed to actual disability. We argue that the preservation of an individual's sociability through enabling nursing approaches, as suggested earlier in this chapter, can diminish or prevent troublesome behaviors. Gray and Stevenson's study (1980) supports this assertion. Individuals with cognitive impairment who shouted and fought with others showed improved behavior and increased verbal interaction following participation in a resocialization group. Other studies have shown that a focus on socialization and accepted social mores (for instance, having control in certain situations) can positively elicit and reinforce socially acceptable behaviors in elders both with and without cognitive impairment (Aasen, 1987; Bernier & Small, 1988; Fates, Smasal, & Betes, 1989; Winger & Schirim, 1989).

In practice, however, enhancing social abilities is not always a priority. Armstrong-Ester and Browne (1986) surveyed 118 nurses on a geriatric unit to elicit their priorities in care and found that patient–nurse communication was a low-level priority. On observation of interactions between nurses and patients, it was noted that nurses spent significantly less time interacting with confused elders than with nonconfused persons. If nurses do not intentionally interact with older people who have cognitive impairment, the social skills of these elders are not used, and other less socially acceptable forms of behavior may be employed for seeking attention and having needs met. When the human need for social contact exceeds environmental stimulation, the person may need to create their own stimulation. In some cases, the behavior may be normative; in others, it may be regarded as disturbed.

There are a few studies that provide guidance to nurses interested in providing environmental stimulation that does not exceed the older person's stress threshold. One example is relaxation training. Two groups of 25 people with Alzheimer's disease were compared on the Stockton State Hospital Geropsychiatric Profile (SSHGP) and participated in a program for one hour, three times a week over a three-month period (Welden & Yesavage, 1982). Individuals in the control group received a group discussion and refreshments. Those in the experimental group received relaxation training, which consisted of self hypnosis, relaxing music, shifting attention from one part of the body another, visual imagery, and refreshments. There was significantly greater improvement on all subscales of the SSHGP for those in the experimental group, whereas the control group showed a slight decline. Two subscales of this measure are social interaction and psychiatric symptoms of a behavioral nature. This study indicates that relaxation training constitutes an environmental stimulation that does not threaten the stress threshold of the older person with cognitive impairment.

Schwab, Rader and Doan (1985) describe a similar program which demonstrates the value of particular types of environmental stimulation for social behavior. The four components of this program are 1) gentle exercise, 2) a vitality or fun component, 3) walking time, and 4) a massage and relaxation component. All but the walking components of this program are accompanied by music. Anecdotal reports of the response of older individuals with dementia to this program include cessation of psychotropic drug use, and of noisy disruptive behaviors. An appropriate social environment can provide the opportunity for experiencing mastery and its companion—enhanced self-esteem.

Cleary, Clamon, Price, and Shullaw (1988) evaluated the effectiveness of a reduced stimulation unit on the abilities of older persons with Alzheimer's disease. The purpose of this unit was to reduce the level of environmental stimulation and to minimize reliance on memory by using specific environmental controls and providing positive and caring interactions. Visual aspects of the unit were a neutral design and color. There was no stimulation from televisions, radios and telephones. Caregiver and visitor access to the unit was controlled. Family and professional caregivers received education in intervention techniques and reduced stimulation. Residents of the unit were permitted free ambulation and received a consistent routine of rest and small group activities. Residents were also permitted to eat and rest where they wished. Attending behaviors and avoidance of the word "no" were encouraged on the part of the caregivers. For the 11 individuals with cognitive impairment who resided on this unit, there was a significant improvement on measures of activities of daily living, and a significant reduction in the behavioral disturbance of agitation and in restraint use. An unanticipated result was an increase in social interaction between the cognitively impaired individuals themselves and between these residents and caregivers. This suggests that it is compensating to remove distracting and burdening environmental stimuli, so that dormant social as well as self-care abilities can be reactivated.

A more individualized approach to ensuring that environmental stimuli do not exceed the stress threshold of the individual may be accomplished through a systematic analysis of behavior (Kline, 1986). Documentation and description of the occurrence of catastrophic behaviors, as well as of events or situations prior to such behaviors, is undertaken. Interventions to reduce or contravene these events or situations are implemented and evaluated. This approach is assistive in establishing congruence between an individual's level of competence and environmental stimulation.

These various programs offer nurses creative ways of offsetting behavioral disturbances that interfere with sociability. They are also compensatory for individuals with Alzheimer's disease who have a lowered stress threshold.

• CONCLUSION •

The sociability of older persons may be threatened as a result of Alzheimer's disease, or as a consequence of excessive or inappropriate environmental stimulation. The numerous social ability-enhancing and ability-compensating approaches that have been described in this chapter can contribute to the quality of life and social experience of these persons.

• REFERENCES •

Aasen, N. (1987). Interventions to facilitate personal control. *Journal of Gerontological Nursing, 13*(6), 21–28.

Adasiak, J. P. (1989). Humor and the Alzheimer's patient: the psychological basis. *The American Journal of Alzheimer's Care and Related Disorders and Research, 4*(4), 18–21.

Alessi, C. A. (1991). Managing the behavioral problems of dementia in the home. *Clinics in Geriatric Medicine, 7*(4), 787–801.

Allen, M. E., Yanchick, V. A., Cook, J. B., & Foss, S. (1990). Do drugs affect social behavior in the confused elderly? *Journal of Gerontological Nursing, 16*(12), 34–39.

Armstrong-Ester, C. A., & Brown, K. D. (1986). The influence of elderly patients' mental impairment on nurse-patient interaction. *Journal of Advanced Nursing, 11,* 379–387.

Bergman, R. (1986). Nursing the aged with brain failure. *Journal of Advanced Nursing, 11,* 361–367.

Bernier, S. L., & Small, N. R. (1988). Disruptive behaviors. *Journal of Gerontological Nursing, 14*(2), 8–13.

Burns, A., Jacoby, R., & Levy, R. (1990). Psychiatric phenomena in Alzheimer's disease. IV: Disorders of behavior. *British Journal of Psychiatry, 157,* 86–94.

Clair, A. A., & Bernstein, B. (1990). A comparison of singing, vibrotactile and nonvibrotactile instrumental playing responses in severely regressed persons with dementia of the Alzheimer's type. *Journal of Music Therapy, 27*(3), 119–125.

Clark, E. (1980). Semantic and episodic memory impairment in normal and cognitively impaired elderly adults. In L. Obler & L. A. Martin (Eds.), *Language and communication in the elderly,* (pp. 47–57). Lexington, MA.: Lexington Books.

Cleary, T. A., Clamon, C., Price, M., & Shullaw, G. (1988). A reduced stimulation unit: Effects on patients with Alzheimer's disease and related disorders. *The Gerontologist, 28*(4), 511–514.

Cohen-Mansfield, J., Marx, M. S., & Rosenthal, A. S. (1989). A description of agitation in a nursing home. *Journal of Gerontology, 44*(3), 77–84.

Dastoor, M. A. (1975). A psychogeriatric assessment program. I. Social functioning and ward behavior. *Journal of Geriatric Society, 23*(10), 465–470.

Dawson, P. (1992). Humor and cognitive impairment. *Perspectives, 16*(1) 2–6.

Fates, M., Smasal, M., & Betes, B. J. (1989). Behavioral psychological intervention. *Journal of Gerontological Nursing, 15*(1), 25–28.

Francis, G., & Baly, A. (1986). Plush animals—do they make a difference? *Geriatric Nursing, 7*(3) 140–142.

Girling, D. M., & Berrios, G. E. (1990). Extrapyramidal signs, primitive reflexes and frontal lobe function in senile dementia of the Alzheimer type. *British Journal of Psychiatry, 157,* 888–893.

Glynn, N. J. (1986). The therapy of music. *Journal of Gerontological Nursing, 12*(1), 6–10.

Goffman, E. (1961). *Asylums.* Garden City, N.Y.: Doubleday.

Gray, P., & Stevenson, J. S. (1980). Changes in verbal interaction among members of resocialization groups. *Journal of Gerontological Nursing, 6*(2), 86–90.

Haley, W. E., Brown, S. L., & Levine, E. G. (1987). Family caregiver appraisals of patient behavioral disturbance in senile dementia. *Clinical Gerontologist, 6*(4), 25–34.

Hall, G. R., & Buckwalter, K. C. (1987). Progressively lowered stress threshold: A conceptual model for care of adults with Alzheimer's disease. *Archives of Psychiatric Nursing, 1*(6), 399–406.

Hendy, H. M. (1987). Effects of pet and/or people visits on nursing home residents. *International Journal of Aging and Human Development, 25*(4), 279–291.

Hoffman, S. B., Platt, C. A., Barry, K. E., & Hamill, L. A. (1985). When language fails: Nonverbal communication abilities of the demented. *Senile Dementia of the Alzheimer Type: Neurology and Neurobiology, 18,* 49–64.

Huff, F. J., Becker, J. T., Belle, S. H., Nebes, R. D., Holland, A. L., & Boller, F. (1987). Cognitive deficits and clinical diagnosis of Alzheimer's disease. *Neurology, 37,* 1119–1124.

Hutchinson, J. M., & Jensen, M. (1980). A pragmatic evaluation of discourse communication in normal and senile elderly in a nursing home. In L. Obler & M. Albert (Eds.), *Language and communication in the elderly.* (pp. 59–73) Lexington, MA: Lexington Books.

Joslyn, D., Grundvig, J. L., & Chamberlain, C. J. (1978). Predicting confabulation from the Graham–Kendal Memory-for-Designs Test. *Journal of Consulting and Clinical Psychology, 46*(1), 181–182.

Kline, K. B. (1986). Systematic data collection: The key to behavioral assessment. *Perspectives, 10,* 4–8.

Kongable, L. G., Buckwalter, K. C., & Stolley, J. M. (1989). The effects of pet therapy on the social behavior of institutionalized Alzheimer's clients. *Archives of Psychiatric Nursing, 3*(4), 191–198.

Langland, R. M., & Panicucci, C. L. (1982). Effects of touch on communication with elderly confused clients. *Journal of Gerontological Nursing, 8*(3), 152–155.

Lawton, M. P., & Nahemow, L. (1973). Ecology and the aging process. In C. Eisdorfer & M. P. Lawton (Eds.), *The psychology of adult development and aging* (pp. 619–674). Washington: American Psychological Association.

Millard, K. A. O., & Smith, J. M. (1989). The influence of group singing therapy on the behavior of Alzheimer's disease patients. *Journal of Music Therapy, 26*(2), 58–70.

Norberg, A., Melin, E., & Asplund, K. (1986). Reactions to music, touch and object presentation in the final stage of dementia: An exploratory study. *International Journal of Nursing Studies, 23*(4), 315–323.

Peter, L., & Dana, B. (1982). *The laughter prescription: How to achieve health, happiness and peace of mind through humor.* New York: Ballantine Books.

Pirozzolo, F. J., Christensen, K. J., Ogle, K. M., Hansch, E. C., & Thompson, W. G. (1981). Simple and choice reaction time in dementia: Clinical implications. *Neurobiology of Aging, 2,* 113–117.

Porszt-Miron, L., Florian, M., & Burton, J. (1988). A pilot study on the effect of rapport on the task performance of an elderly confused population. *Canadian Journal of Occupational Therapy, 55*(5), 255–258.

Posner, M. I., & Boies, S. J. (1971). Components of attention. *Psychological Review, 78*(5), 391–408.

Ripich, D. N., & Terrell, B. Y. (1988). Patterns of discourse cohesion and coherence in Alzheimer's disease. *Journal of Speech and Hearing Disorders, 53,* 8–15.

Rosendahl, P. P., & Ross, V. (1982). Does your behavior affect your patient's response? *Journal of Gerontological Nursing, 8*(19), 572–575.

Schwab, Sr. M., Rader, J., & Doan, J. (1985). Relieving the anxiety and fear in dementia. *Journal of Gerontological Nursing, 11*(5), 8–15.

Sullivan, J. L., & Deane, D. M. (1988). Humor and health. *Journal of Gerontological Nursing, 14*(1), 20–24.

Swearer, J. M., Drachman, D. A., O'Donnell, B. F., & Mitchell, A. L. (1988). Troublesome and disruptive behaviors in dementia: Relationships to diagnosis and disease severity. *Journal of the American Geriatrics Society, 36*(9), 784–790.

Tennant, K. F. (1990). Laugh it off. The effect of humor on the well-being of the older adult. *Journal of Gerontological Nursing, 16*(12), 11–17.

Teri, L., Larson, E. B., & Reifler, B. V. (1988). Behavioral disturbance in dementia of the Alzheimer's type. *Journal of the American Geriatric Society, 36*(1), 1–6.

Webster's Ninth New Collegiate Dictionary. (1987). Springfield, MA: Merriam-Webster.

Winger, J., & Schirim, V. (1989). Managing aggressive elderly in long term care. *Journal of Geriatric Nursing, 15*(2), 28–33.

Welden, S., & Yesavage, J. A. (1982). Behavioural improvement with relaxation training in senile dementia. *Clinical Gerontologist, 1*(1), 45–49.

Witte, K. (1987). Discourse and dialogue: Prolonging adult conversation in the Alzheimer patient. *American Journal of Alzheimer's Care and Research, 3*(1), 30–40.

FOUR

INTERACTIONAL ABILITIES

A CENTRAL ELEMENT OF NURSING IS THE INTERPERSONAL relationship. Within this relationship, the nurse comes to understand the individual's needs, hopes and desires, and the subjective meaning of the health or illness experience to the individual. Together, the nurse and person share values and negotiate plans regarding care. For this kind of relationship to emerge, both nurse and individual rely on verbal and nonverbal language that we call interactional abilities. These abilities enable us to express our ideas and to understand what the other person is attempting to communicate. When interactional abilities are compromised, individuals may be at risk of social isolation (Dawson, Kline, Crinklaw-Wiancko, & Wells, 1986). Lee (1991) reports that communication difficulties are among the most common problems facing family members when caring for individuals with dementia.

Interactional abilities are affected by dementia. It is known that general and specific language changes occur with dementia and that these changes are present in all stages of the disease (see, e.g., Appell, Kertesz, & Fisman, 1982; Bayles, 1982; Bayles & Tomoeda, 1991; Becker, Huff, Nebes, Holland, & Boller, 1988; Cummings, Benson, Hill, & Read, 1985; Murdoch, Chenery, Wilks, & Boyle, 1987). For someone experiencing language changes, the words of others may sound strange and unfamiliar, it may resemble the experience of visiting a foreign country. To communicate may be a struggle when words or other language symbols become elusive. It is likely to be frustrating and frightening for those living through these changes. It is equally frustrating for the caregiver, as caregiving unfolds within an interpersonal relationship which is heavily dependent on language (Lee, 1991).

• CLINICAL FEATURES AND THREATENED ABILITIES •

The major clinical feature of dementia that affects language is called aphasia, or the language of dementia. Aphasia is described by Pryse-Phillips and Murray (1986) as affecting the comprehension of language and the verbal expression of ideas. Through an understanding of the specific ways in which aphasia affects individuals with dementia, nurses can select and use language purposefully to elicit retained abilities or to compensate for lost interactional abilities.

Aphasia in dementia has been studied by Cummings, Benson, Hill, & Read (1985). Although they studied aphasia for the significance of language to the diagnosis of Alzheimer's disease, their findings have relevance for nursing in that they inform us of abilities threatened by aphasia. In their study, 30 people with senile dementia of the Alzheimer's type who scored below 24 on the Mini-Mental State Exam were compared with 70 healthy spouses or family members who scored above 24 on the Mini-Mental State Exam. On 37 subtests of language function, the healthy control subjects scored zero, which indicated no difficulty, whereas the older people with dementia scored greater than zero, indicating difficulty. The language functions most affected were found to be the information content of spontaneous speech, comprehension of commands, naming, sentence completion, word list generation, writing to dictation, narrative writing, and completion of nursery rhythms. The authors concluded that language abnormalities were present in all patients with Alzheimer's disease, readily distinguishing them from control subjects, including aged controls.

From the Cummings, Benson, Hill, and Read study we learn that the comprehension of language and the verbal expression of ideas are indeed abilities affected by dementia. These findings of difficulty with comprehension and expression of language are similar to those of Appell, Kertesz, and Fisman (1982), Becker, Huff, Nebes, Holland, and Boller (1988), and Murdoch, Chenery, Wilks, and Boyle (1987). The interactional abilities that have implications for caregiving, and that will be discussed in this chapter, include comprehension of verbal commands, reading, naming, sentence completion (word retrieval), the information content of speech (verbal fluency), and writing. We have subsumed these interactional abilities under two main categories: comprehension abilities and expression abilities.

In this chapter, we proceed to examine studies which specifically address these abilities, in order to come to a deeper understanding of the influence of aphasia on language or the interactional abilities of people with dementia. It is of utmost importance that we gain an appreciation of how the interpersonal relationship can be facilitated and sustained between nurses and individuals when language is impaired.

• COMPREHENSION ABILITIES •

UNDERSTANDING OF SENTENCES

"Mr. Jones walks away from me when I talk to him" or "Mrs. Smith becomes restless when I talk to her" are statements caregivers may make that reflect the response of individuals with dementia who have difficulty with verbal comprehension. Why does this individual withdraw when someone is speaking? When there is difficulty with comprehension, language may become a source of burden or high environmental press.

In the introduction to this chapter, aphasia was described as affecting the comprehension of language. Aphasia affects verbal comprehension, which is also referred to in the literature as auditory comprehension. Verbal or auditory comprehension refers to the understanding and processing of information which an individual hears, and has been shown to be affected by dementia (Appell, Kertesz, & Fisman 1982; Becker, Huff, Nebes, Holland, & Boller 1988; Murdoch, Chenery, Wilks, & Boyle, 1987). The loss of verbal comprehension is progressive in dementia and, over time, increasingly larger portions of what is said is lost by the individual with cognitive impairment. A simple statement like "pick up the wash cloth and wash your face" may be heard differently. The individual may hear and make sense of some of the information in the statement, but the rest may sound like nonsense. For example, the statement may sound like "pick up the shawlthoc and apso, so uyo nac shaw uryo face". The individual may respond by touching her face. This action is appropriate to the portion of the statement understood, but it appears inappropriate within the context of the total command.

The loss of verbal comprehension as a result of aphasia threatens the ability to understand sentences or commands. We have observed that the comprehension of complex sentences will be affected before that of simple sentences. Excess disabilities that may result from this loss are social isolation and withdrawal as a response to spoken language which exceeds the individual's competence.

The findings and methods of a study by Appell, Kertesz, and Fisman (1982) provide information regarding the loss of the ability to understand sentences and instructions, as well as ways in which to determine the level at which an individual can understand information. Twenty-five older people with Alzheimer's dementia were compared with 141 individuals with stroke aphasia and with 24 healthy older persons. Those with Alzheimer's disease scored lower on verbal comprehension than both those with stroke aphasia and the healthy control group. Similarly, Murdoch, Chenery, Wilks, and Boyle (1987) found that the auditory comprehension of 18 older people with Alzheimer's disease was significantly lower than that of 18 institutionalized, non-neurologically impaired control subjects.

It is noteworthy, however, that within verbal comprehension there was greater ease in the understanding of some sentences than others for individuals with Alzheimer's disease (Appell et al., 1982). The understanding of yes/no sentences was easier than the understanding of sentences with sequential commands.

The ability to follow sequential commands refers to the ability to obey commands of increasingly complex sentences (Kertesz & Poole, 1974). A one-part command consists of one verb and one noun. "Touch your nose" is an example. A two-part command consists of two verbs and two nouns, such as "Clap your hands, and point to the window;" and a three-part command contains three verbs and three nouns, for example, "Touch your knee, close the book, and shut your eyes."

Yes/no sentences are sentences to which either yes or no is an appropriate response. "Will a stone sink in water?" or "Does it snow in July?" are examples of yes/no sentences (Kertesz & Poole, 1974). Also, yes/no sentences are sentences that are composed of common knowledge and either infer or state a comparison. For example, the sentence "Is summer hotter than winter?" asks a question which is based on common knowledge and provides a comparison.

Individuals with cognitive impairment secondary to Alzheimer's disease have difficulty with respect to verbal or auditory comprehension, and this difficulty may vary with the complexity of language. The above studies are helpful in determining where an individual is on the continuum of language comprehension loss.

METHOD OF ASSESSMENT

The loss of verbal comprehension in dementia is progressive; therefore, we want to determine the level of the older person's comprehension ability within their range of understanding from complex, to simple, to yes/no sentences. This assessment is accomplished by the use of sequential commands and yes/no sentences.

The older person is asked to follow one-part commands relating to self and to objects. Self-related commands are those which are specific to the individual, such as "Touch your nose" or "Close your eyes." Object-related commands require that the individual direct attention beyond their self to the immediate environment. "Point to the ceiling" or "Hand me the book" are examples of object-related commands. In our assessments we have found that the ability to understand self-related commands will be retained sometimes even when there is a loss of ability to understand object-related commands. When the individual demonstrates a comprehension of one-part commands, the assessment progresses to two-part commands. Self-related and object-related two-part commands are given. An example of a self-related two-part command is: "Stamp your feet and then close your eyes;" an object-related two-part command is: "give me the pen then point to the window." When two-part commands are understood, the individual is asked to follow three-part commands. A simple three-part command, consisting of one verb in combination with three nouns, precedes a more complex command of three verbs and three nouns. An example is the following: "Pick up the pen, pick up the cloth, then pick up the spoon," followed by "Point to my face, raise your arms, then clap your hands."

Common knowledge and fixed choice questions requiring either a yes or no answer are asked of the older person to determine comprehension of yes/no sentences. A response of yes or no, respectively, to the questions "Does Tuesday come after Thursday?" or "Are cars faster than airplanes?" indicates that the sentences have been understood. The assessment of verbal comprehension begins with yes/no sentences, as individuals with cognitive impairment have less difficulty in understanding yes/no sentences than sequential commands. Nevertheless, we understand, as Hier, Hagenlocker, and Shindler's (1985) work indicates, that older persons with dementia have greater difficulty in responding to yes/no sentences than those without dementia.

Nursing Actions

Ability Enhancing

Nursing actions which are ability-enhancing for older persons who have retained verbal comprehension abilities are:

1. the matching of language complexity with the competence of the individual;
2. speaking at a normal rate, pace, and voice tone;
3. the use of abstract or concrete language consistent with the individual's competence,
4. the selection of group activities according to the individual's language competence.

If the language used in interaction with an individual with cognitive impairment is of greater complexity than the individual's understanding, language becomes a source of high stimulation, and may burden the individual. Conversely, if an individual has a verbal comprehension level which is greater than the complexity of language used, stimulation may be low, and there may be further loss of comprehension simply through disuse. The goal is always to match language complexity with the competence of the individual.

Once the level of verbal comprehension is known, sentences are sequenced in interactions with individuals to enable the person to retain that level of ability as long as possible. Sentences are purposely formulated to the level of one, two, or three parts in interaction. This requires that the nurse be very conscious of how she uses language. It also ensures that environmental stimulation matches competence. In our practice, for example, a gentleman was reported to show intermittent agitation or aggression. On assessment, it was found that he was able to respond to one- and two-part commands. When presented, however, with three-part commands, he became upset and agitated. This behavior demonstrates how complexity of language greater than the individual's competence can be a source of high stimulation.

It is also important to speak at a normal rate, pace, and voice tone, regardless of the level of sentence complexity. Clear enunciation and short pauses between words assist the individual to hear and process the words. Speaking in louder tones and with long pauses between words distort what is being said and interfere with the individual's ability to understand (Nebes, Boller, & Holland, 1986). Through an appropriate sequencing of sentences, interactional abilities are consistently reinforced. Interaction can then be a source of experiencing success, an experience often eluding the individual with cognitive impairment.

The response of an individual to sequential commands also influences the kind of language a nurse uses to be ability-enhancing. When an individual understands three-part commands and therefore complex sentences, we have found in practice that the use of abstract language as well as concrete language may be understood in interactions. In other words, interaction may be conducted in a normative fashion. But when the understanding of an individual is limited to one- or two-part commands, the nurse selects more concrete language in order to enhance the older person's ability to comprehend. This approach is ability-enhancing, as there is a more pronounced loss of comprehension for abstract than for concrete language (Appell, Kertesz, & Fisman, 1982; Murdoch, Chenery, Wilks, & Boyle, 1987).

The response of an individual to one-, two- and three-part commands also helps the nurse to determine the context in which interaction will be enhancing to the individual. For example, if an individual understands three-part commands, we have found that group interactions which focus on language-related activities, such as discussions of current events or support groups, can be relevant. For individuals who understand only one- or two-part commands, group activities which focus on music or exercise may be more appropriate, as they are less language dependent. Verbal interactions are encouraged to maintain this level of comprehension, but take place on a one-to-one basis.

NURSING ACTIONS

Ability Compensating

When older persons have lost verbal comprehension abilities, nursing actions are selected that are ability-compensating. These are:

1. the use of yes/no and open-ended sentences;
2. the use of nonverbal language;
3. awareness of personal and the older person's body language;
4. direct physical assistance.

The first approach to compensate for the loss of the ability to understand sequential commands is to use yes/no sentences, provided that the assessment demonstrated retention of this ability. When an individual understands yes/no sentences, open-ended questions are posed which help the elder to convey her needs. "Are you thirsty?", "Are you hungry?" and "Are you in pain?" are ways to learn the needs of the individual who has lost comprehension of complex language. The use of open-ended questions can also help to evaluate the effectiveness of our care. For instance, inquiring about the individual's comfort or asking "Does this help?" while giving an intervention can afford the individual the opportunity to provide feedback regarding our nursing actions.

Nonverbal language is used to compensate for the loss of verbal comprehension. If an individual can still imitate, as indicated in the self-care assessment, then demonstration can be used to provide guidance to the individual in conducting daily activities. Also, awareness of our own body language and facial expression, and the need for congruence between them, is important in communicating purposefully to the individual with cognitive impairment. Further, touch in combination with single words such as "eat" while stroking the forearm (as discussed in the self-care chapter) can compensate for verbal language loss and facilitate successful completion of an activity.

A severe loss of the ability to comprehend language necessitates providing direct physical assistance to the individual and protecting the individual from excessive stimulation and noise in the proximal environment. As well, it is important to be aware of the older person's facial expressions and body language, which may convey positive and negative responses to our interactions (Hoffman, Platt, Barry, & Hamill, 1985). Documentation of these non verbal responses is required so that all people providing care are consistent in their interpretation and approach. This eliminates a trial-and-error method of caregiving, and, simultaneously, the risk of inducing too much environmental stimulation.

The world is probably a very strange and uncomfortable place when words no longer convey meaning. Attention to comfort measures and to being present with the individual in a nonthreatening way are critical in sustaining the interpersonal relationship. The therapeutic strength of a smile is inestimable. In the chapter on social abilities it was shown that elders with severe cognitive impairment are still responsive to the emotional undertones in the environment. Thus, nursing actions that convey a positive intent are compensating for individuals with cognitive impairment.

READING COMPREHENSION

Nurses may observe that an individual with cognitive impairment can read with ease, but cannot use this information in a meaningful way. What might explain this response to written words?

Aphasia, which affects the comprehension of both verbal and nonverbal language, interferes with the ability of an individual to understand, and eventually to read written words (Murdoch, Chenery, Wilks, & Boyle, 1987). Appell, Kertesz, and Fisman (1982) found that reading comprehension presents greater difficulty than verbal comprehension. In their study, individuals with cognitive impairment scored 4.6/10 on follow-through of verbal commands, but only 3.1/10 on reading and follow-through of written commands. Therefore, it is anticipated that an individual who has lost verbal comprehension may also have difficulty with reading comprehension.

Although the ability to understand what is written may be lost, the ability to read aloud or word-reading ability may be retained for a long period of time (Cummings, Houlihan, & Hill, 1986; Nelson & O'Connell, 1978). In the Cummings, Houlihan, and Hill study, reading comprehension was assessed by the recognition of words and nonwords, comprehension of written commands, and understanding sentences. The ability to discriminate words and nonwords was present to some extent in all individuals. However, the ability declined in those with lower mental status scores. The same pattern was observed with respect to understanding commands and sentences. Nine of 13 individuals could read aloud more commands than they could understand. Although the ability to understand written words declines with the advancing of dementia, the ability to read is preserved, and can serve as a means for older persons with cognitive impairment to experience success.

The ability to read aloud is probably related to the ability to recognize words. Clarke (1980) has found discrimination of words and nonwords to be relatively well-preserved in spite of cognitive impairment. Clarke compared cognitively impaired individuals with healthy older persons and college students regarding their ability to recognize words and distinguish words from nonwords. In her study, all individuals were asked to press a yes/no button when presented with a word or a nonword. The individuals with dementia were able to distinguish between words and nonwords as easily as the elders without illness and the college students. The only difference was in the speed of response; the ill older persons took longer than the two comparison groups. Similarly, in another study, the ability to recognize written words as belonging to categories was equivalent for older persons with dementia and for healthy older controls (Huff, Corkin, & Growdon, 1986). Through these studies, we gain an insight into the effect of aphasia both on reading comprehension ability in older people with dementia and more generally, word-reading ability but without comprehension.

METHOD OF ASSESSMENT

Sequential commands similar to those used in the assessment of verbal comprehension are employed to assess reading comprehension. First, one-, two-, and three-part written commands are visually presented on a cue card, and the older person is requested not to read the command out loud, but rather to carry out the command. This clearly establishes reading comprehension ability. Then the individual is asked to read aloud the command, which indicates reading ability but not necessarily comprehension. The information gained from this assessment is useful in deciding what kinds of memory aids will be assistive to the individual.

NURSING ACTIONS

Ability Enhancing

Nursing approaches that are ability-enhancing for individuals who retain reading comprehension ability are:

1. the use of written memory aids;
2. creation of opportunities for reading;
3. audiology consult to ensure optimal hearing levels.

Written memory aids provide guidance and structure to the experience of the individual when the ability to read with comprehension is retained. The complexity or amount of written information that is given to an individual is ability-enhancing when it matches the individual's demonstrated level of reading comprehension. Retention of the ability to understand one- or two-part written commands means that simple written memory aids, such as the ordering of activities in the day or directional word signs to guide ambulation, are ability-enhancing. When an individual understands three-part written commands, this level of comprehension is preserved by providing books or magazines of interest.

If individuals are able to read aloud, reading aloud to another person will be ability-enhancing as well as providing an experience of success. In the book *The Memory Board* by Jane Ruhl (1987), an older woman with Alzheimer's disease reads to a blind man. An individual with cognitive impairment can still reach out and provide a meaningful experience for another human being.

It may be found on assessment that an individual understands written better than verbal commands. If this is so, referral to an audiologist is indicated, because there should be less difficulty with spoken than with written language as stated above. An individual with a diagnosis of dementia whom we assessed was found to respond to complex written commands with ease, but he had been unable to follow through on verbal commands. Following an audiology consultation and the subsequent receiving of a hearing aid, his performance in all activities increased significantly and the diagnosis of dementia was removed from his chart. Individuals with dementia who have greater difficulty with verbal comprehension than reading comprehension can also increase their abilities following an audiology consultation and provision of a hearing aid.

NURSING ACTIONS

Ability-Compensating

Ability-compensating nursing approaches are employed for older persons with dementia who have lost reading comprehension ability. These are:

1. the use of familiar symbols and personal belongings;
2. the use of semantically related words to assist with comprehension;
3. the consistent and frequent use of verbal reminders.

Written memory aids are not useful when reading comprehension has been lost. A woman whose name was written on her door reported that the name on the door was that of a nurse who worked there part-time. For this woman written information was of no value. However, a picture of her husband at her bedside helped her to find her personal space and identify where she belonged. Familiar symbols and personal belongings (when their recognition has been assessed and found to be retained) can be compensating for the individual when written memory aids are no longer useful. Because they are a form of abstraction, it is important to note that symbols as memory aids be familiar, so that the older person is not over-burdened.

In order to provide opportunities to experience success to the person who has lost the ability to comprehend written information, lists of words and nonwords can be used in creative ways as a diversional activity. For example, reading words aloud, facilitated by using a semantically related word such as "doctor" to precede the word to be read such as "nurse" (Nebes, Martin, & Horn, 1984) is a possible recreational activity. As well, frequent and consistent verbal reminders can be used as memory aids, rather than written information; for example, reminding the person every 15 minutes that lunch will be in one hour. When we are providing compensating actions for the individual who has lost the ability to comprehend written information, we look both to the environment and to our verbal interactions to make up for this lost ability.

• EXPRESSION ABILITIES •

On occasion, each one of us has experienced difficulty accessing an exact word or words, or naming an object or person. Although such occasions can be frustrating for us, we are usually soon relieved when the word or words we require to interact verbally or in writing promptly appears in our consciousness. But, for individuals with aphasia, the words that they require to interact in a meaningful way or to accurately express their needs, wants and preferences are not always recoverable. Their ability for verbal or written expression has been radically altered in the presence of Alzheimer's disease. Therefore, it is completely comprehensible that these individuals may become frustrated and at times agitated, and that they are always at risk for excess disability in terms of maintaining human interaction and relationships and being understood by others.

Length of stay in an institution has been found to be associated with the decline of several major language functions (Appell, Kertesz, & Fisman 1982; Holland, cited in Murdoch, Chenery, Wilks, & Boyle, 1987), which may be a consequence of the progression of the disease. But it may also reflect excess disability that can arise in relation to caregivers' lack of appreciation of language function in individuals with Alzheimer's disease. Murdoch et al. (1987) found that length of stay was not correlated with a decline in major language functions with the exception of articulation. The objective for nurses is to come to an understanding of how the individual's expression abilities have altered, in order to design ways of continuing meaningful interaction and interpersonal relations in the course of day-to-day caregiving and daily living for the person.

The behavior of individuals observed in clinical practice, and the general and research literature on dementia (see, e.g., Appell, et al., 1982; Murdoch et al., 1987; Nebes, Boller, & Holland, 1986; Pryse-Phillips & Murray, 1986) confirm that a problem with verbal and written expression exists. For instance, in practice, we have frequently heard nurses or the family of afflicted individuals state that they had difficulty comprehending what the person wanted. The person may state "I want that," and when asked "What," they may repeat "That," and if provided with the incorrect item, the person may become angry. Difficulty with verbal expression may be poorly understood by nurses and can make nursing care intricate. In the following section, we discuss several studies which are helpful in illuminating the nature of verbal and written expression changes with dementia. These studies provide a guide for caregiving when they are interpreted for nursing practice.

OBJECT IDENTIFICATION

The ability to name or to identify objects verbally has been found to be more difficult for elders with Alzheimer's disease than for persons with other diseases and/or for normal subjects (Bayles & Tomoeda, 1983; Becker, Huff, Nebes, Holland, & Boller, 1988; Huff, Corkin, & Growdon, 1986; Martin & Fedio, 1983). For example, naming was found by Bayles and Tomoeda to be a problem for 62% of moderately impaired Alzheimer's individuals. What is note-worthy is that 38% of Alzheimer's subjects with moderate impairment and all the mildly affected individuals were found to retain the ability to name, which supported an earlier finding by Bayles and Boone (1982). Also, although Alzheimer's subjects were likely to misname, the misnaming was often semantically associated with the test item (Bayles & Tomoeda, 1983), a finding of other researchers (Martin & Fedio, 1983). That is, the actual object to be named was replaced with a word that had a similar meaning. Huff, Corkin, and Growdon, (1986) suggest that the inability to name is not due to a lack of recognition of the object, but rather to difficulty with word retrieval.

In terms of daily living, loss of naming with aphasia threatens the person's ability to label what she wants. The individual may not be able to specify and express needs, wants and feelings or to interact with others in an understandable manner. Hence, the assessment of naming ability or what we call "verbal object identification" is an important part of the enablement nursing process.

METHOD OF ASSESSMENT

Several of the previously mentioned studies have been helpful in developing our approach to assessment. Generally speaking, in the literature, subjects are given a confrontation naming task, which includes a series of pictures. They are asked to look at and name the object in the picture. For our assessment of verbal object identification, we present familiar objects. Familiar objects are selected because they represent concrete articles which the older person encounters in day-to-day living. Also, the object is presented within view or held by the person as this facilitates identification (Appell et al., 1982). The individual is asked to verbally identify the object and the nurse records whether the response is correct, related to the object presented, or incorrect.

NURSING ACTIONS

Ability Enhancing

The following nursing approaches are ability-enhancing when the person retains language expression abilities:

1. the use of verbal specificity in communication;
2. the placement of objects within the visual field;
3. listening for semantic relatedness in communication;
4. the provision of adequate time for responses.

When an individual retains the ability to verbally identify an object, the nurse encourages verbal specificity during interaction to preserve use of the ability. For example, when the individual says "I want that," the nurse prompts her to name the desired object. To facilitate an individual's verbal expression, objects are placed within her visual field, or she is allowed to hold the object.

In each interaction, the nurse listens closely for semantic relatedness, because this implies some meaningful object recognition. For example, the individual may say "pen" when attempting to say "pencil." Or, while the actual word description may be lost, the object function (e.g., hair grooming) is retained. Above all, allow the individual time to find the precise word required to express himself. Persons with dementia have been found to require more time than normal individuals to name objects, especially objects whose names are unfamiliar (Lawson & Barker, 1968, cited in Bayles, 1982).

Nursing Actions

Ability Compensating

Nurses can use the following ability-compensating actions when language expression abilities are lost:

1. define and describe the relevant item needed for care;
2. the use of cues using semantically related words;
3. name the suspected item of interest for the individual.

When the ability for verbal object identification is lost, the nurse can provide definitions of items that the individual seems to be requesting or attempt to uncover the name of the object to which the person is referring. For example, if it is suspected that the individual is trying to say the word "glass," the nurse can respond by saying "Is it something that you drink from?" Or conversely, she can ask the individual to describe what she wishes or feels, if naming is a problem. Martin and Fedio's (1983) research suggests that individuals with word-finding problems, which was found to be correlated with inability to name (Huff, Corkin, & Growdon, 1986), are often able to describe their intent.

Nurses may also assist the person to find a word or words by cueing them with semantically related words, which Nebes, Martin, and Horn (1984) call semantic primes. For instance, if the person is attempting to say the word "comb," the word "brush," which has a similar meaning, can be used as a prime. Also, phonemic prompts can be compensating. These are words which sound the same. For instance, suggesting "blood pressure" when the person has said "blad prussion" is a phonemic prompt. The phonology of most words in individuals with dementia is correct or nearly correct (Bayles, 1982), so by attending closely to the individual's verbal expression and/or offering appropriate phonological cues, purposeful interaction can continue.

When definitions or semantic and phonemic primes are ineffective, then it is compensating for the nurse to name prosthetically by the employment of force/choice questions. For instance, the question "Would you like an apple, an orange or a banana?," supplemented by placing these objects within the visual field of the person, may facilitate the successful expression of her needs.

The individual may be able to demonstrate the use of the object when she has lost the ability to name it (Schwartz, Marin, & Saffran, cited in Appell et al., 1982). If so, assess the individual's ability to gesture or demonstrate object use, such as that of a pen or a cup, and if this ability is retained, ask the individual to demonstrate the purpose of the object. Also, by naming the object for the individual at opportune moments, such as mealtime, the nurse can help the individual to relate items to words. These actions serve to continue a sense of interpersonal interaction and facilitate the routines of everyday living.

WORD-RETRIEVAL ABILITY

In addition to naming difficulties, a problem with verbal expression in the presence of dementia may include an inability to select a particular word. The specific ability at risk for the individual is the finding of a word or words needed to communicate one's wishes or needs, and generally to make oneself understood in interpersonal communication.

Nebes, Boller, and Holland (1986), in their study of the effect of semantic context on the performance of individuals with Alzheimer's disease, found, among other results, that word finding or the ability to retrieve words was less difficult when sentence context was highly constrained. That is, there was substantially less difference between dementia and normal subjects when the sentence context restricted the range of possible responses to a few items. The researchers labelled this type of sentence a "high cloze" sentence.

A high cloze is one in which the range of possible endings of the sentence is limited. "Cats see well in the _____ (dark)" is an example of a sentence in which both the context and an acceptable choice of words to complete it is circumscribed. "The mouse ran up the _____ (clock)" is another example of a high cloze sentence, whereas "he left the room and _____ (?)" is an instance of a low-cloze or much less restrictive sentence. To find a word or words to complete a low-cloze sentence is obviously more difficult. In fact, both young and older normal individuals take longer to complete low-cloze sentences than they do high-cloze sentences (Cohen & Faulkner, 1983, cited in Nebes et al., 1986). Also, older persons with dementia make fewer errors on high cloze sentences than on low cloze sentences (Nebes et al., 1986). Therefore, to assess the ability of an individual with dementia to retrieve or find words, it is best to employ high-cloze sentences, and to select those sentences that are not peculiar to culture or educational level.

METHOD OF ASSESSMENT

The individual is asked to complete a short sentence in which the final word is missing. The sentence is read to the individual. Advise her that it is a single word that makes sense that is required to complete the sentence. Sentences such as those that follow are appropriate to the assessment:

1. Roses are red, violets are _____.
2. They fought like cats and _____.

3. Christmas comes in the month of _____.
4. The grass is _____.

If the individual responds appropriately to the latter (third and fourth) sentences, then repeat the former sentences. Individuals with cognitive impairment may need the opportunity to learn the task prior to evaluation. Responses which are usual or make sense are acceptable. Additionally, allowing enough time to recover the word is important, as it takes these individuals a much longer time than normal persons to word-find.

Nursing Actions

Ability Enhancing

The ability to retrieve words is enhanced by these nursing approaches:

1. the use of high-cloze sentences;
2. the use of low-cloze sentences when this ability is retained.

In caregiving, when the ability to retrieve words is present, it is important to employ high-cloze sentences, which can partially offset the word-finding problem in individuals with dementia, and facilitate word retrieval and possibly their own decisionmaking (Nebes et al., 1986). A highly bounded context might be achieved by saying "For shaving you will use a _____ . . ." However, it may not be necessary to restrict interaction to high cloze sentences for these individuals who retain the ability to word-find. Low-cloze sentences can be used also in interactions for those individuals who are able to recover words in broader sentence contexts. But this higher level of interpersonal interaction must be monitored closely, so as not to overwhelm the individual and create excess disability in terms of her ability to retrieve words and complete interactions. As a diversional activity, one could have a list(s) with high-cloze sentences, thereby engaging the individual in interaction.

NURSING ACTIONS

Ability Compensating

When the ability for word retrieval is lost, appropriate ability-compensating approaches are:

1. assuming the major responsibility for interaction,
2. the use of sentences requiring yes/no responses only.

If an elder has lost the ability to complete highly restricted sentences, as determined on assessment, then the caregiver may need to assume the greater responsibility for interaction. Rather than expecting an individual to complete an interaction with a specific word or words, we might ask questions that require yes or no responses only. Conversely, the nurse may wish to initiate and/or complete the interaction, or include other basic nonverbal interactional techniques to enhance the interaction. All of these approaches are designed to compensate for this particular language deficit while maintaining interpersonal communication.

ABILITY TO DESCRIBE

Aphasia in dementia can also imperil one's ability to use language creatively (Bayles, 1982; Martin & Fedio, 1983), or to convey meaning in discourse (Appell et al., 1982; Hier, Hagenlocker, & Shindler, 1985; Kempler, Curtiss, & Jackson, 1987; Murdoch et al., 1987), while syntactical or grammatical ability (Kempler, Curtiss, & Jackson, 1987) and the ability to articulate (Murdoch et al., 1987) may be preserved. In caring for cognitively impaired older persons, it may be noticed that their speech lacks meaning or substance, although it is correct grammatically. Information content is missing (Cummings, Benson, Hill, & Read, 1985). These persons seem unable to put together a series of related ideas; one idea does not appear to connect with another. There is the intention to communicate but an inability to conceptualize what is to be said. Bayles (1982) draws an analogy between this behavior and computers which mechanically print a message like "garbage" as a consequence of a problem in the software program. Appell et al. (1982) refer to this type of spontaneous speech in dementia persons as circumlocution and semantic jargon: "Speech may be verbose and circuitous, running on with a semblance of fluency, yet incomplete and lacking coherence. Examination of content shows the speech to be in many cases vague, meaningless, incoherent, or unintelligible" (p. 74). Hier et al. (1985) note that as the disease progresses, speech becomes even more disintegrated, but that in the earlier stages verbal fluency, or what we call the ability to describe, is maintained to some extent. This latter finding is not consistent with Martin and Fedio's (1983) research. They found fluency abilities to be affected in mildly impaired individuals with suspected Alzheimer's disease.

On qualitative analysis of the spontaneous speech of a sample of 25 Alzheimer's patients, Appell et al. (1982) discovered a high incidence of semantic jargon. While grammar was preserved, much of the speech was irrelevant and the meaning lost; the speech had lost its communicative purpose. Similarly, Hier et al. (1985) found on quantitative analysis of a picture description task that the speech of dementia subjects compared to normal subjects was empty, that is, fewer total words and unique words were used. Additionally, these persons failed to make relevant observations. Individuals who are more severely affected are least able to use language to convey information. Kempler, Curtiss, and Jackson (1987) found similarly, in their analyses of spontaneous speech, that syntactical construction was preserved while there was poor lexical or vocabulary use. When the ability to describe is jeopardized, there is difficulty verbally describing daily life events, which has implications not only for communication with others, but also for safety. Persons so affected are simply less able to convey or obtain information, or to direct their own or the actions of others. In order to identify and preserve verbal fluency abilities and compensate for the loss of ability to communicate information, careful assessment is required.

Method of Assessment

In order to assess the ability for verbal fluency, a simple but systematic approach is to ask the individual to describe the room he or she is in (Pryse-Phillips & Murray, 1986). The retention of this ability is indicated when the individual describes the contents of the room using a reasonable number of words possessing conciseness and fairly accurate meanings, as well as the use of complete sentences or an appropriate use of nouns and verbs. The ability to describe is found to be lost verbal when either response is attempted but no meaningful description is provided or when there is no verbal response.

Nursing Actions

Ability Enhancing

In order to preserve the ability to describe, older persons with dementia are:

1. engaged in regular and frequent interactions;
2. presented with open-ended questions.

As is the case when other interactional abilities have been found to be present, ability-enhancing nursing actions include encouraging verbal interaction. The promotion of verbal fluency might be accomplished by way of regular and frequent conversation, or the inclusion of dementia individuals in verbal discussion groups. The use of open-ended questions and fostering questioning by the individual is another effective way of stimulating verbal fluency in conversation. Friedman and Tappen (1991) provide another creative method of increasing or maintaining verbal fluency in older persons with Alzheimer's dementia. In their study, conversing with individuals while walking significantly improved verbal fluency as compared to individuals who were engaged only in conversation. This intervention is important to both expression abilities and mobilization. The authors suggest that in times of cost constraint, planned walking plus conversation is a less costly intervention and one that can be undertaken by families and nonprofessionals.

NURSING ACTIONS

Ability Compensating

Ability-compensating nursing approaches for the individual who has lost the ability to describe are:

1. creating the opportunity for individuals to engage in singing;
2. the encouragement of automatic language.

When the ability to describe is lost, the person is encouraged to sing or to use "automatic" language. The latter refers to highly familiar language used mostly in social contexts. As an illustration, the nurse might say "Isn't it a nice day" or "How are you" with the goal of inspiring some verbal interaction and discouraging social isolation. Singing is another way of evoking automatic or highly familiar language. It is not uncommon to observe older persons with the aphasia of dementia singing familiar songs.

Also, it is important and appropriate to promote interaction between individuals similarly affected with aphasia. On several occasions, we have noticed residents with cognitive impairment engaged in verbal interaction with one another. Although no meaningful content was identifiable, there was certainly a reciprocation of words and expression occurring between these individuals. The need for human interaction will endure regardless of the state of language competencies.

WRITING ABILITIES

Written expression may be lost in the presence of dementia (Cummings, Benson, Hill, & Read, 1985; Murdoch et al., 1987), and often perishes prior to oral language abilities (Appell et al., 1982), and early in the disease process (Allison, 1962; Gustafson, Hagberg, & Ingvar, 1978; Sjogren, Sjogren, & Lindgren, 1952 cited in Appell et al., 1982). As can be imagined, the inability to express oneself in writing has a multitude of implications inclusive of strain with instrumental tasks, such as jotting reminders down of upcoming events and managing one's financial matters, and with more interpersonal activities, including the writing of letters to loved ones or writing for personal pleasure.

METHOD OF ASSESSMENT

The assessment of the ability to write is similar to the assessment of the ability to verbally identify an object. Three to four familiar objects are presented and the individual is asked to write both the name of the object and its use. Writing ability is considered present when the individual is able to successfully perform these tasks; it is considered to be absent when the individual cannot fulfill this request. Difficulty with penmanship may be observed. This is more reflective of excess disability than loss of the ability to express oneself in writing.

NURSING ACTIONS

Ability Enhancing

When writing ability is retained, nurses can suggest letter writing, consistent with the person's lifestyle, or other applications of writing as a diversional activity. For example, as the writing of names may be a retained ability (Murdoch, Chenery, Wilks, & Boyle, 1987), these individuals may assist with preparing name lists for unit or ward activities.

Nursing Actions

Ability Compensating

When the ability to write is lost, then the nonwritten expression abilities explained above are fostered, as they are likely to be retained longer than written abilities (Appell et al., 1982). Further, the nurse may assume the responsibility of performing writing tasks for the individual.

• Conclusion •

The language changes associated with dementia are pervasive. However, general assumptions cannot be made regarding an individual's language competencies or the nursing approaches to be taken. Through an understanding of the interactional abilities which are threatened by aphasia in dementia, nurses can purposefully assess individuals to determine which abilities have been retained or lost. The knowledge gained in the assessment process guides nurses to select or develop approaches that are specific to the individual, either enhancing retained abilities or compensating for lost abilities. The Enablement Nursing Process ensures that individuals with cognitive impairment continue to participate in human relationships, which is fundamental to the personal life experience and to the practice of nursing.

• References •

Appell, J., Kertesz, A., & Fisman, M. (1982). A study of language functioning in Alzheimer patients. *Brain and Language, 17,* 73–91.

Bayles, K. (1982). Language function in senile dementia. *Brain and Language, 16,* 265–280.

Bayles, K., & Boone, D. (1982). The potential of language tasks for identifying senile dementia. *Journal of Speech and Hearing Disorders, 47,* 210–217.

Bayles, K., & Tomoeda, C. (1991). Caregiver report of prevalence and appearance order of linguistic symptoms in Alzheimer's patients. *The Gerontologist, 31*(2), 210–216.

Bayles, K., & Tomoeda, C. (1983). Confrontation naming impairment in dementia. *Brain and Language, 19,* 98–114.

Becker, J., Huff, J., Nebes, R., Holland, A., & Boller, F. (1988). Neuropsychological function in Alzheimer's disease. *Archives of Neurology, 45,* 263–268.

Clark, E. (1980). Semantic and episodic memory impairment in normal and cognitively impaired elderly adults. In L. Obler and L. A. Martin (Eds.), *Language and communication in the elderly* (pp. 47–57). Lexington, MA: Lexington Books.

Cummings, J., Benson, F., Hill, M., & Read, S. (1985). Aphasia in dementia of the Alzheimer type. *Neurology, 35,* 394–397.

Cummings, J. L., Houlihan, J. P., & Hill, M. A. (1986). The pattern of reading deterioration in dementia of the Alzheimer type: Observations and implications. *Brain and Language, 29,* 315–323.

Dawson, P., Kline, K., Crinklaw-Wiancko, D., & Wells, D. (1986). Preventing excess disability in patients with Alzheimer's disease. *Geriatric Nursing, 7*(6), 299–301.

Friedman, R., & Tappen, R. M. (1991). The effect of planned walking on communication in Alzheimer's disease. *Journal of the American Geriatrics Society, 39*(7), 650–654.

Hier, D., Hagenlocker, K., & Shindler, A. (1985). Language disintegration in dementia: Effects of etiology and severity. *Brain and Language, 25,* 117–133.

Hoffman, S., Platt, C., Barry, K., & Hamill, L. (1985). When language fails: Nonverbal communication abilities of the demented. *Neurology and Neurobiology, 18,* 49–64.

Huff, J., Corkin, S., & Growdon, J. (1986). Semantic impairment and anomia in Alzheimer's disease. *Brain and Language, 28,* 235–249.

Kempler, D., Curtiss, S., & Jackson, C. (1987). Synactic preservation in Alzheimer's disease. *Journal of Speech and Hearing Research, 30,* 343–350.

Kertesz, A., & Poole, E. (1974). The aphasia quotient: The taxonomic approach to measurement of aphasic disability. *The Canadian Journal of Neurological Sciences, 1*(1), 7–16.

Lee, V. (1991). Language changes and Alzheimer's disease: A literature review. *Journal of Gerontological Nursing, 17*(1), 16–20.

Martin, A., & Fedio, P. (1983). Word production and comprehension in Alzheimer's disease: The breakdown of semantic knowledge. *Brain and Language, 19,* 124–141.

Murdoch, B., Chenery, H., Wilks, V., & Boyle, R. (1987). Language disorders in dementia of the Alzheimer type. *Brain and Language, 31,* 122–137.

Nebes, R., Boller, F., & Holland, A. (1986). Use of semantic context by patients with Alzheimer's disease. *Psychology and Aging, 1*(3), 261–269.

Nebes, R., Martin, D., & Horn, L. (1984). Sparing of semantic memory in Alzheimer's disease. *Journal of Abnormal Psychology, 93*(3), 321–330.

Nelson, H. E., & O'Connell, A. (1978). Dementia: The estimation of premorbid intelligence levels using the new adult reading test. *Cortex, 14*, 234–244.

Pryse-Phillips, W., & Murray, T. J. (1986). *Essential neurology* (3rd ed.). New York: Medical Examination Publishing Company.

Rule, J. (1987). *Memory board.* Tallahassee, FL: Naiad Press

FIVE

INTERPRETIVE ABILITIES

I N NURSING, WE UNDERSTAND THAT HUMAN BEINGS ARE CON-
stantly engaged in a dynamic interaction with the environment, and that our practice focus is the human response to the
environment (Carpenito, 1989). This response may be affected by a
person's interpretive abilities. Interpretive abilities are those competencies that allow us to derive meaning from the external world:
the world of people, objects, and events. Additionally, interpretive
abilities enable us to assess our own internal environment or inner
feeling states.

In the presence of progressive dementia, interpretive abilities
may be threatened. The external world may appear foreign and
threatening as people, objects and events no longer convey the same
meaning, as was illustrated earlier in the imaginative journey. At
the same time, there is a potential for inner feeling states to be
affected by dementia. Catastrophic behaviors may be a response to
an increasingly burdensome environment, as suggested by the con-

cept of environmental press. From an enabling perspective, nurses might suspect that these behaviors reflect excess disability, possibly arising in the process of caregiving when we fail to understand interpretive abilities and dementia, and the relevant nursing approaches.

The clinical features of dementia that have impact on interpretive abilities are recognition deficits, which include prosopagnosia; diminished recognition of emotion; astereognosis; disorientation to time; memory deficits; and depression. These specific clinical features of dementia affect the interpretive abilities of recognition of self and familial others, recognition of emotion, recognition by touch, recognition of time, recall ability, and the ability to experience pleasure (subjective feeling states).

• RECOGNITION •

ABILITY TO RECOGNIZE SELF AND FAMILIAL OTHERS

CLINICAL FEATURES AND THREATENED ABILITIES

"Mrs. Brown is frightened by her own face in the mirror," and "Mother doesn't recognize me anymore" are common statements made by those involved in the caregiving of older people with dementia. Both Mrs. Brown and the speaker's mother fail to recognize very familiar faces. It is unclear whether the ability to recognize is due to impairment in retrieval (recall) of information or in storage of information, but the net result is the same: an inability to recall well-rehearsed information (Sainsbury & Coristine, 1986). The term for this clinical feature of dementia is prosopagnosia, which is defined as the inability to recognize the faces of known people (Pryse-Phillips & Murray, 1986).

The first clinical description of prosopagnosia dates to the turn of the century and was given by Lord David Cecil. Lord Cecil relates the following story:

The fifth marquess of Salisbury (intermittently Prime Minister of Britain) found it hard to recognize the faces of his fellow men, even his relations, if he met them in unexpected circumstances. Once, standing behind the throne at a court ceremony, he noticed a young man smiling at him. "Who is my young friend?" he whispered to a neighbor. "Your eldest son," the neighbor replied (Damasio, Damasio, and Van Hoesen, 1982).

Confirming Lord Cecil's anecdotal description, Wilson, Kaszniak, and Fox (1981) studied the ability of older persons with cognitive impairment to recognize famous faces. In their study, 20 older people with cognitive impairment were compared with 24 healthy individuals regarding their recognition of the faces of people famous between 1920 and 1975. The people with cognitive impairment recognized significantly fewer famous faces than the healthy individuals. The failure of individuals with cognitive impairment to recognize the familiar faces of their own family members can be distressing to the family causing feelings of isolation and concern regarding the value of continued interactions or visits.

Another study by Sainsbury and Coristine (1986) tested whether some form of recognition is retained by individuals with moderate to severe dementia with respect to family members. They selected 15 individuals who failed to recognize pictures of close relatives who had visited in the past week. Each individual was asked to look at four Polaroid pictures. One of the pictures was that of a close relative who had recently visited. The other pictures were of strangers matched for age and sex. The individual was first asked if they recognized any of the pictures. Recognition was assumed even if the subject picked out the picture of the relative but could not remember the relative's name. If recognition did not occur, the subject was asked to choose one picture that they liked better than the others. They predominantly chose the picture of the relative. So while these individuals could not identify or recognize pictures of close relatives, they chose the picture of the relative in response to a preference request.

The authors concluded that while conscious recognition may not be present, another form of memory still remains, which they call "affective memory." Sainsbury and Coristine make this link on the basis of the individuals' correct response to the directive "choose the picture that you like better." They speculated that the source of the response may have come from either simple familiarity, or from affective or emotional association. There may be value, then, in continuing family contact.

For some individuals with cognitive impairment, failure to recognize oneself in a mirror may be experienced. We assessed 40 older persons with moderate to severe dementia with respect to this ability and found that 11 of these individuals were unable to identify themselves in the mirror. Forstl, Burns, Jacoby, and Levy (1991) report that only 7 of 128 persons with Alzheimer's dementia misidentified themselves in a mirror. The majority of persons probably retain self recognition ability.

The presence or absence of the ability to recognize oneself in a mirror influences caregiving. When recognition of self in the mirror is absent, mirror images may be sources of increased or meaningless stimulation. When it is present, the mirror can provide feedback during caregiving activities and reinforce self-identity.

METHOD OF ASSESSMENT

This is assessed by asking the older person to identify herself in either a mirror or a photograph, and by asking the person to read her own name and indicate whose name it is. Self-recognition is present if the individual responds positively on either of these assessments. The ability is lost when no recognition for self occurs.

NURSING ACTIONS

Ability Enhancing

Nursing actions that are ability-enhancing for individuals who have retained the competency of self recognition consist of:

1. the use of a mirror for feedback and positive reinforcement of self;
2. the use of name signs to identify personal space;
3. the assessment of picture preference;
4. the use of family and personal photographs in reminiscence.

Hygiene and grooming activities can be enhanced by the use of a mirror. Although we have not studied this, our clinical observations suggest that increased participation and interest in self-care is afforded through the feedback of a mirror. Small successes or evidence of mastery can be conveyed in this simple way.

When persons can recognize their written name, personal belongings and space can be identified and marked through name signs. This can be reassuring to individuals with cognitive impairment.

When the ability to recognize oneself is present but family members indicate that they are not recognized, the continued ability to *affectively* recognize a family member in a picture becomes vital information for the family. Preference of pictures which contain family members is then assessed. If the ability is found to be present, the information is shared with the family, who may find this both encouraging and comforting. This may also motivate family members to continue visiting older persons with cognitive impairment who are institutionalized. Nurses are cautioned not to jump to conclusions when the spouse says "My husband doesn't recognize me; he consistently thinks our daughter is me." The person may recognize the face of the wife at a younger age in the face of the daughter, and may, in fact, be making a correct identification. Although this may be distressing to the family member, the person is usually making positive affective associations with the spouse.

NURSING ACTIONS

Ability Compensating

When the ability to recognize self and familial others is lost, it is compensating to:

1. cover mirrors;
2. teach family about the significance of clothing and voice tones.

Catastrophic reactions can occur if the older person is suddenly confronted with an unknown face in a mirror (even her own). Rather than curtail activities that normally occur in rooms that have mirrors, the approach of choice is to cover the mirror so that these activities can continue to be performed in an environment that is as close to normal as possible. Hygiene should occur in the bathroom rather than at the bedside. By compensating for the loss of this interpretive ability, we can prevent excess disability in relation to self-care.

Whiteley and Warrington (1977) have contributed to our understanding of what interventions are possible when all ability to recognize familiar faces is lost, including affective recognition. They found that recognition was enhanced by other characteristics when facial recognition was lost, namely, the presence of other visual materials such as clothes and voice tones. Wearing familiar clothes and engaging in conversation, then, may be ability compensating.

RECOGNITION OF EMOTION

CLINICAL FEATURES AND THREATENED ABILITIES

Failure of an individual with cognitive impairment to respond to the tears or sadness of a loved one, or to the anger of a co-resident in a long-term care facility, may indicate a loss of recognizing facially expressed emotions. The clinical feature here is diminished recognition of emotion or prosopo-affective agnosia, and has been identified by Kurucz, Feldmar, and Werner (1979). Diminished recognition of emotion is defined as impairment in the ability to recognize affect, and is believed to be a function of cognitive decline, and not the result of a primary impairment of perception of emotion (Albert,

Cohen, & Koff, 1991). This clinical feature of dementia threatens the person's ability to recognize facial affect such as sadness, happiness and anger, and therefore, to identify the feeling state of others.

In their study, Kurucz, Feldmar, and Werner (1979) tested 3 groups of 14 elders for their responses to happy, sad, and angry facial expressions. One group had dementia, one group other psychiatric diagnoses, and the third group was normal. They found that only the group with dementia demonstrated difficulty with the recognition of emotion. Those with dementia made errors in the identification on all facial expressions, particularly the expression of anger (51% error rate).

The perception of affect recognition has been studied by Albert et al. (1991). Comparing 19 residents with Alzheimer's dementia and 19 residents without cognitive deficits, the investigators found that those with dementia had significantly more difficulty labelling emotions on people's faces. They also had greater difficulty in selecting the correct emotion to correspond with facial expression when the verbal labels were provided by the examiner. These studies suggest that there is a risk of harm for older persons who have lost the ability to recognize emotion. Facial expressions are normally strong cues for withdrawing from a threatening situation; if the person does not recognize emotion, she may not understand when a harmful situation is imminent.

METHOD OF ASSESSMENT

To assess the ability to recognize facial affect, the nurse shows the individual three pictures of facial emotions. The pictures convey happy, sad, and angry facial expressions. As each facial expression is presented, the nurse asks: "Tell me if she is happy, sad or angry." If verbal comprehension ability is lost, the assessment can be done using a yes/no technique: "Is she angry?," "Is she sad?," "Is she happy?" Correct responses indicate that the ability is retained for recognizing affect.

Nursing Actions

Ability Enhancing

An ability-enhancing action, when the ability to recognize emotion is present, is to convey congruence between facial and verbal expression on the part of the nurse.

When individuals retain the ability to recognize the feelings of others, congruence between verbal and nonverbal language is important. For example, the wife of a gentleman with dementia would verbally convey that everything was all right, but was upset and worried about another situation in her life. Her nonverbal communication was incongruent with her verbal communication. During and following her visits, her husband became restless and anxious. When she acknowledged her sadness and worry, he was able to console and comfort her through hugging her and stroking her hand. He then remained calm during and following her visits.

Nursing Actions

Ability Compensating

When individuals are unable to discern emotion through facial expression, ability-compensating nursing actions are:

1. accentuate body posture when conveying affective information;
2. verbally describe emotions;
3. teach family members about the loss of facial affect recognition and alternate ways to convey emotional information, as per 1) and 2);
4. protect the individual from potentially harmful situations.

The study of Brosgole, Kurucz, Plahovinsak, Sprotte, and Haveli-wala (1983) is assistive in planning ability-compensating nursing actions in the presence of prosopo-affective agnosia (PAA). These authors found that affect or feeling may be more readily recognized through body posture than through facial expression. They examined the responses of 8 men and 8 women with Alzheimer's dementia to: (1) photographs of faces, (2) caricatures of faces, (3) animal caricature faces, and (4) postural drawings, all of which conveyed affective expressions of happy, sad, and angry. The results indicated that the elders with dementia were more able to read the postural expression of emotion than facial expressions, and that they were much more able to interpret the facial expression of happiness than the sad or angry faces.

When the ability to recognize facial affect is absent, the nurse assumes a compensating role. Prosthetic techniques, such as verbally describing and posturally portraying feeling states, are used. Everyone in the environment is alerted to the fact that the individual has difficulty in recognizing emotion, and is reminded to be constantly vigilant for threatening situations that may not be recognized by this individual.

RECOGNITION BY TOUCH

CLINICAL FEATURES AND THREATENED ABILITIES

Tactile object discrimination, or the ability to recognize objects by touch, is an interpretive ability. It is important for self-care in relation to recognizing and using buttons, zippers, fasteners, combs, and brushes. We have found that the ability to recognize by touch was present in only 51% of 40 individuals with moderate to severe dementia. Astereognosis is the inability to recognize common objects by touch. As a consequence, older persons with astereognosis may be unable to obtain information about objects.

METHOD OF ASSESSMENT

The assessment of the ability to recognize objects by touch is adapted from de Leon, Potegal, and Gurland (1984). The individual is instructed to close her eyes and identify by touch four small objects placed in her hand such as a key, a ring, a safety pin, and an elastic band. In a second test, two cups of different sizes are placed one in each hand, and the person is asked to identify the hand holding the larger cup.

When the person is able to identify any of the small objects, the ability to recognize by touch is present. If only the identification of the smaller or larger cup is present, then recognition ability by touch is limited to that of the size of the object. Recognition of objects by touch is considered to be absent when no correct responses to the assessment are observed.

NURSING ACTIONS

Ability Enhancing

When recognition by touch is present, it is ability enhancing to:

1. supplement verbal guidance with tactile cues;
2. provide a "rummage" box as a diversion.

Recognition by touch can be used to facilitate self-care. Allow the person to hold objects that you are talking about, such as a knife when guiding the person to prepare their food. As well, the ability to recognize by touch can be used as a diversionary tactic for those individuals known to actively seek stimulation by rummaging through the drawers of coresidents. A rummage box can be provided with a variety of tactile stimulation that might include zippers, buttons, clasps and fasteners.

Nursing Actions

Ability Compensating

It is ability-compensating for the individual who has lost the ability to recognize by touch to provide verbal and visual cues.

Visual and verbal cues required to compensate for the lack of tactile recognition might consist of the following: guide the hand to the zipper, direct the person's gaze to the zipper, and state "close the zipper." Alternatively, velcro closures might be assistive if they are familiar to the older person.

RECOGNITION OF TIME

Clinical Features and Threatened Abilities

Clocks and calendars are used as time markers to enable us to manage and anticipate life's daily events. They guide us in decisions about when to eat, dress, sleep, meet, go to work, remember events, and anticipate seasonal weather changes. The early literature on cognitive impairment unanimously supported the use of these environmental props for older persons with a progressive dementia, and they served as a backbone for reality orientation therapy. We now know that the ability to relate to these props in a meaningful way may be impaired with dementia. The older person is at risk for excess disability when she is challenged to use or recall time when the ability is not present; human competency and the environment are not matched, and withdrawal may result.

The work of Shulman, Shedletsky, and Silver (1986) is helpful in determining the extent to which the ability to recognize time remains intact. These authors established that appropriate clock drawing is a useful adjunctive screening instrument for cognitive impairment that is free of cultural and educational bias. In their study, subjects were given a pre-drawn circle and asked to set the time at three o'clock. This would include drawing both the numbers and the hands appropriately. Shulman and his group identified that the degree of decline of cognitive impairment correlated positively with the decline in ability to draw the clock.

Calendars are the other time marker that should be considered in terms of their usefulness for caregiving. In our assessment of 30 individuals with cognitive impairment, 55% retained the ability to recognize calendar time.

METHOD OF ASSESSMENT

We assess for the ability to recognize clock time by illustrating two clock faces: one representing on the hour time, and the other, hour and minute time (see Figure 5.1).

Recognition of calendar time is assessed by showing a monthly calendar and asking the person to: (1) point to two dates identified by the nurse, (2) read out loud two dates pointed to by the nurse.

NURSING ACTION

Ability Enhancing

To promote the continued use of existing abilities with respect to time when found to be present in the assessment, it is useful to have:

1. clocks and time cues in the proximal environment;
2. a daily schedule at the bedside;
3. significant events marked on a calendar.

Clocks can be a valuable aid to promote orientation. When older persons are able to read time, ensure that clocks are always within the visual environment. Structure the day using hours and minutes

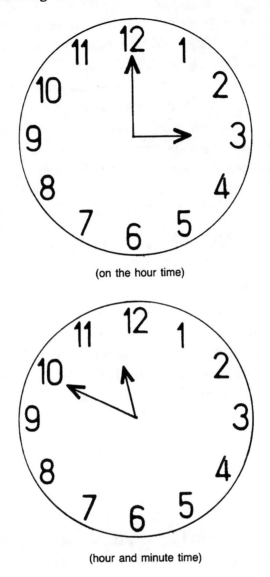

(on the hour time)

(hour and minute time)

Figure 5.1
The two clocks, one representing hour time, and the other representing hour and minute time, are used to assess the ability to recognize clock time.

and use time-related interactional statements and questions to reinforce this competency. For example, "What time do you go for exercise?" "It is 10:30." When the ability to read time by the hour only is present, structure the day with hourly markers, and similarly use only hourly time related statements and interactions.

A digital watch has been reported as ability-enhancing for a gentleman with a mild dementia (Kurlychek, 1983). By beeping every hour, the alarm reminded the gentleman to check the notebook in which he kept track of his daily program in the hospital.

When the ability to use calendars is present, they can be used as a cue for daily orientation, activities and upcoming events, seasons, or family visits. Nurses in long-term care facilities who work with individuals with cognitive impairment have no doubt found that the marking of family visits on a calendar can be a source of providing reassurance to these individuals. Questions about family are asked repeatedly by some older people with dementia. We have found that when we point to the present and the visit dates on the calendar, the older person will cease asking questions for a while. Because of memory decline, this may have to be repeated, but providing information in this manner has a calming effect for at least short periods.

Nursing Actions

Ability Compensating

Actions which are compensating when the interpretive ability to recognize time is lost are:

1. the use of general time markers;
2. acceptance of individual's sense of time.

General time markers such as morning, afternoon, lunch, and bedtime are used to provide some orientation to time. Similarly, period markers such as the season or Christmas, rather than the specific month and date, are provided. Reality orientation to person, place, and time is no longer meaningful (Gubrium & Ksander, 1975; Mattice & Mitchell, 1990)!

When recognition of time is lost, the time frame to which the individual is relating is accepted, rather than orientation to real time being encouraged (Feil, 1992). For the nurse, the only focus in the present time is on establishing a trusting and supportive relationship with the older person. Following Feil (1992), some of the techniques to accomplish this include listening with empathy and exploring the content of the older person's communication using questions—"who, what, where, when and how," and repeating of words to the older person.

RECALL ABILITY

CLINICAL FEATURES AND THREATENED ABILITIES

As dementia progresses, the ability to recall or remember progressively declines. Both recent memory and remote memory are affected, although the former loss occurs at an earlier phase (Reisberg, 1983). Memory loss has impact on multiple abilities in the daily living experience, from forgetting new information just learned to information that is more entrenched, such as the names of close family and friends.

Although the extent and rate of memory loss differs from person to person, it is nevertheless anxiety-provoking, and may result in feelings of fear and denial, as was illustrated in the imaginative journey. Environmental props and intentional interactions on the part of the nurse are extremely important and assistive in reducing the accompanying anxiety and related behaviors.

Throughout the lifespan, remote and recent memory provides us with a background from which to interpret and derive meaning in the experience and events of day-to-day living. Relating to situations in daily living can present a tremendous challenge for individuals with cognitive impairment. Nurses can offer these individuals assistance in meeting this challenge by understanding the effect of dementia on the interpretive ability of recall.

Several studies have examined remote and recent memory in older persons with dementia. In some of these, remote memory has been the focus of interest. Twenty older persons with dementia were compared with 24 healthy individuals on tests of memory by Wilson, Kaszniak, and Fox (1981). The older persons with dementia had greater difficulty remembering persons and events famous between 1925 and 1975 than the healthy older persons. Of the persons and events presented, half were classified as "easy to remember" and half as "hard" or "more difficult." The people with dementia did not differ significantly from the healthy group on the "hard" questions. But the older persons with dementia had significantly greater difficulty answering the easy questions. The older persons with dementia also had greater difficulty remembering persons and events from the remote past than the healthy individuals. Similarly, Kopelman found that 16 persons with Alzheimer's disease had greater difficulty recalling remote news events and famous personalities than 16 healthy older persons (Kopelman, 1989). However, those with Alzheimer's disease did recall events of earlier decades more often than those in recent decades, while more recent events were recalled with greater ease by the healthy subjects.

In Kopelman's (1989) study, autobiographical and personal facts about the past were studied with respect to remote memory. The individuals with Alzheimer's disease remembered more from their early childhood and early adult period than from recent years, although they still remembered less in comparison to the healthy older people. For those with Alzheimer's disease, the scores on autobiographical (61%) and personal facts (75%) were much higher than for news events (30% or less).

Fromholdt and Larsen (1991) also studied autobiographical memory by asking 30 older people with cognitive impairment to tell about the events that had been important in their lives. The older people with cognitive impairment had greater difficulty in recalling events in all time periods than the 30 healthy older persons in the control group. But they recalled relatively more from adolescent and early adult periods. We learn from these studies that the remote memory of persons with dementia is impaired in comparison with healthy older persons, and that for persons with dementia, personal recollections are easier to retrieve from earlier life periods than the recent past.

Memory for category names versus item-specific names has also been studied by researchers, and provides some insight into the nature of information more easily recalled. Mr. Jones is able to remember that apples are fruit, although he can't remember the word "apple." This suggests that object categories can be used to facilitate interpretation. Martin and Fedio (1983) found that 14 older persons with Alzheimer's disease were able to recall category meaning more easily than item—specific names. When asked to recall items found in a supermarket, those with dementia provided category names such as fruits, vegetables, and meats rather than more specific items such as apples, carrots, and beef. To extrapolate these findings to caregiving, using categories and cues may be more helpful than item—specific names.

In support of Martin and Fedio, Nebes, Boller, and Holland (1986) found no difference between older persons with dementia, normal older people, and the young in their ability to place words into categories. Knowing that an elder is still able to make category associations can be very helpful to the caregiver, who can then intentionally offer category choices whenever possible by saying for example: "Get dressed," rather than "Put on your shirt."

The recent memory of older persons with dementia had been studied using lists of words and pictures of unfamiliar faces (Diesfeldt, 1990; Eslinger & Benton, 1983; Miller, 1975; Wilson, Kaszniak, Bacon, Fox, & Kelly, 1982; Wilson, Kramer, Fox, & Kaszniak, 1983). Typically, the individual is presented with words or pictures one at a time and is asked to recall the words. Later, words or pictures presented initially are interspersed or paired with new words or faces. The person is asked to indicate which of these words or pictures were previously seen. Persons with dementia have greater difficulty in recalling words or faces than persons with other neurological deficits or than healthy controls. Recent memory for both words and faces is difficult for persons with Alzheimer's disease, except when the words or faces are highly familiar. From these studies, we learn that familiar words or information may be recognized with greater ease than unfamiliar information, but that overall recall is diminished.

To summarize, the abilities threatened in the presence of recall, or memory deficits associated with a progressive dementia are: (1) the ability to recall items and events from the past (remote memory), (2) the ability to recall categories and item-specific names, and (3) the ability to remember recently given information recent memory).

METHOD OF ASSESSMENT

The F.A.C.T. test (Issacs & Kennie, 1973) is used to assess recall. It has the advantage over other dementia screening tools of identifying not only memory ability, but also the ability to categorize. In this test, described by Gallo, Reichel, and Andersen (1988), the nurse asks the older person to name as many items as she can, up to 10 in each of four categories: fruits, animals, colors, and towns (F.A.C.T.). The test is not timed.

A deficit of memory is indicated by the inability to recall items. In our assessment of 40 older persons, we found that about 30 percent of them were able to recall some information in each category. Recall of any of the items suggests some ability and the recognition of categories.

NURSING ACTIONS

Ability Enhancing

When some recall or memory abilities are present, as indicated by a score of two or three per category, it is ability-enhancing to incorporate into caregiving:

1. memory training techniques, such as partial information, spaced retrieval, and encoding and visual image associations;
2. autobiographical reminiscences.

Providing partial information, such as the initial letters of a word, has been demonstrated to improve recall (Miller, 1975; Morris, Wheatley, & Britton, 1983). As a game, recall abilities can also be enhanced by asking individuals to recall words when given the initial letters of the word: "fruits that start with A" for example; and to point to objects within a given category and within the environment, such as pictures, chairs, and people.

To assist individuals to remember, spaced retrieval shows promise as an ability-enhancing approach. Abrahams and Camp (1991) have shown improvement in the memory ability of two older women using this approach, which involves repetition of information at ever-increasing time intervals. A target item, such as a word, is named and the individual is immediately requested to repeat the word. Five seconds later, the individual is asked to recall the word. When the individual is successful after five seconds, the interval period is increased. With each successful recall, time intervals are lengthened. Over time, the two women who received this approach were able to recall a word or item after a period of several days. This approach is described anecdotally as useful in day-to-day living situations by Arkin (1991). She relates that her mother, who suffers from Alzheimer's disease, would ask a question repeatedly. Upon giving her mother the answer, Arkin asked her to remember the answer for 30 seconds. The interval was increased to one minute, then five minutes, and at ongoing increased intervals. After five hours, the information continued to be retained. In practice, we often see individuals who ask the same question over and over. Through providing follow-up to the question at spaced and increasing intervals, specific information may be retained.

Encoding has also been described as ability enhancing for recall (Rosswurm, 1989). While the person is viewing a stimulus, the nurse describes attributes of the stimulus or object, such as its color and shape. Rosswurm reports that 21 older persons with Alzheimer's disease improved their recall scores by 90% after receiving encoding cues, namely, "The orange is round and orange, and can be eaten."

Visual image associations, such as photographs with large print labels, are recommended by Geiger (1988). These can be used in retraining individuals to recall caregivers' names.

Reminiscences of autobiographical information from earlier life periods can be encouraged (Kopelman, 1989; Fromholdt & Larsen, 1991). The nurse, either in one-to-one situations or in group contexts, asks members to talk about earlier times: school days, marriages, and significant humorous/sad experiences. Opportunities for individuals to exercise some of their memory ability in regard to personal and other information can contribute to experience of success and mastery.

Nursing Actions

Ability Compensating

When recall abilities are diminished, as indicated by a score of one or zero, ability compensation is accomplished through the use of:

1. external memory aids;
2. category context with visual cues;
3. environmental supports;
4. audio and visual tapes.

External memory aids can be ability-compensating. As discussed in the chapter on interactional abilities, written memory aids can be useful when reading comprehension abilities are present. Other external memory aids, such as timers, calculators, and activity charts as suggested by Geiger (1988), may be tried, but their success will depend on the presence of other interpretive and interactional abilities: time recognition, and reading abilities.

The nurse uses category context in combination with visual cues to assist in comprehension. Show the elder person the washcloth and say "This is for washing," or show three fruits to the person and ask "Which fruit would you like to eat?" For individuals who have minimal recall ability, active participation in reminiscence groups is not ability-compensating. However, the environment and activities can be structured in other ways to evoke familiar past activities or memories, such as singing, dancing, cooking, and/or food aromas.

According to Arkin (1991), audio- and videotapes of familiar people and family events can provide comfort and reassurance when recall abilities are absent. Earlier in this chapter, we learned that affective memory, as demonstrated by preference of family members' pictures, may be present when recall and recognition memory are compromised.

SUBJECTIVE FEELING STATES

CLINICAL FEATURES AND THREATENED ABILITIES

A person's ability to relate to and derive pleasure from the surrounding environment is influenced by personal feelings. The ability to express and interpret feelings is another interpretive ability. Being able to express personal feelings of boredom, anxiety, worry, and sadness can enable a person to seek help when appropriate, or to express dissatisfaction with a current situation. An inability to express these feelings can lead to their intensification and to demoralization or depression. Caregivers may overlook the negative feeling states because of the language deficits and the diminished facial expression that are associated with dementia. Hence, a risk for excess disability of social isolation, withdrawal, boredom, and agitation may arise.

Recent studies have shown that although it is not readily apparent, persons with a progressive dementia continue to be able to both accurately express and interpret feeling states (Ryden & Knopman, 1989; Martin & Fedio, 1983; Hoffman, Platt, Barry, & Hamill, 1985). The challenge to nurses is to identify and confirm feeling states, and to develop enabling environments that ensure appropriate expression and interpretation.

Initially, we will consider the ability of older persons with cognitive impairment to respond to questions about feeling states. Ryden and Knopman (1989) administered the Philadelphia Geriatric Morale Scale to 56 patients with memory loss who were admitted to their dementia clinic. They found that more than 82% were able to complete the entire measure except for one item.

The work of Martin and Fedio (1983) is supportive of Ryden and Knopman (1989). They serendipitously discovered the same result in their study comparing elders with dementia and normal persons on word production and comprehension of single words. There was no significant difference between the groups on broad category judgements requiring appreciation of feeling states.

The following clinical scenario experienced by one of the authors is illustrative of both of these research papers. Mr. B. is 75 years old. He was diagnosed as having Alzheimer's disease three years ago, and was institutionalized one year ago. At the time of assessment, he was still fully ambulatory, continent with scheduled toileting, and could feed himself, but required considerable assistance with bathing, dressing, and grooming. His language skills were marked by word-finding difficulties, a paucity of vocabulary, and an inability to correctly sequence words and structure sentences. Frequently, he was unable to finish a sentence. Mr. B. was asked yes/no questions that inquired about feeling states, such as happy, sad, and worried. When asked if he experienced boredom, he sat upright in his chair, looked straight in the eye of the nurse and clearly answered, "It's amazing the amount of nothing to do around here." Fortunately, at this time he was being assessed for his potential to participate in an activities group!

Another supporting clinical example of the ability to accurately convey or express feeling states is reported by a colleague (Mitchell-Pederson, 1990). Upon asking an aunt with dementia shortly following her institutionalization, "How are you?" our colleague received the following reply: "I feel that I'm living in a world of strangers and I'm the chief stranger." The poignancy of this example serves to underscore the need to assess for feeling states and to provide appropriate and individualized interventions.

Akerlund and Norberg (1986) demonstrated that elders with dementia who participated in a one-hour psychotherapeutic discussion group that facilitated expressions of loneliness, disappointment, worry, guilt, and illness showed evidence over time of increased verbal activity regarding these feelings and increased interaction with other group members. This study is illustrative of the type of group activity which can enhance the expression of subjective feeling states.

Frequently nurses make observations about the behavior of elders with dementia, and speculate about the cause of feelings, without a systematic assessment. Cohen-Mansfield (1986) illustrated that when a group of nursing home nurses were surveyed for their perceptions of 66 older persons who were exhibiting agitation, they attributed the agitation to subjective feeling states; yet, there was no evidence of systematic assessment for what might be causing the discomforting feelings.

The need for nurses to conduct an assessment of feeling states is critical for providing enabling care, and for the identification of depression. Depression in the elderly is often characterized by signs and symptoms resembling dementia (Gurland & Toner, 1987; Kane, Ouslander, & Abrass, 1989; Wells, 1979) is frequently referred to as pseudodementia. Elders with dementia may experience an accompanying depression. Depression is treatable. A positive response to treatment is usually accompanied by an improvement in the cognitive and functional abilities although the underlying dementia remains.

Depression has been reported in approximately one-quarter of elders who are correctly diagnosed as having dementia (Kral, 1983;

Wands, Merskey, Hachinski, Fisman, Fox, & Boniferro, 1990; Siegel & Gershon, 1987; Jeste & Wragg, 1989). Cummings, Miller, Hill, & Neshkes (1987) found 17% of 30 older persons with Alzheimer's disease and 60% of persons with multi-infarct dementia had scores in the depressed range of the Hamilton Depression Rating Scale. Recent sudden changes in cognition or functional abilities and stated feelings of worry, anxiety, or sadness may be indicators of depression. The nurse is often the first to suspect depression and is therefore in a position to conduct a quick screen and initiate the consultation process.

Depression associated with dementia can be treated pharmacologically. Steele, Rovner, Chase, and Folstein (1990) claim that when a depression superimposed on a dementia is recognized and treated, it might delay or prevent institutionalization of some individuals. This is because the persons' cognitive and functional abilities increase as the depression lifts. Depression here represents a cause of excess disability. Although treatment of depression in dementia is still in its infancy, Wragg and Jeste (1989) support intervention, as this can often improve quality of life for elders and their families.

When depression coexists with dementia or is presenting similarly to dementia, the ability to experience pleasure is threatened.

METHOD OF ASSESSMENT

The purpose of assessing feeling states is to determine if the older person is experiencing positive or negative feelings. If negative feelings predominate, then nurses undertake further assessment with respect to depression.

The resident is asked simple "yes" or "no" questions about her feeling state. There are six feeling states addressed in their assessment. They are: sadness, anxiety, happiness, worry, contentment, and boredom. The nurse simply states, "Mrs. B., I'm going to ask you some questions about how you are feeling." The nurse proceeds to ask the older person to answer "yes" or "no" as to whether or not she has been feeling: (1) sad, (2) anxious, (3) happy, (4) worried, (5) content, or (6) bored. After each question, time is given for the older person to respond before proceeding to the next.

The ability to perceive pleasure is indicated by a "yes" response to the feelings of happiness and contentment, and by "no" responses to sad, anxious, worried and bored. If responses indicate a more negative state of feelings, as indicated by "no" responses to the positive feelings and "yes" responses to the negative feelings, then further assessment with respect to depression is undertaken. This is accomplished by observation of behavior, or by asking specific questions of the person or family regarding cognitive decline. The questions to be asked are: "Has there been a sudden rather than a consistent gradual change in behavior?" "Has there been a rapid rather than a slow progression of cognitive decline?" "Is there variability in performance of tasks of daily living or is performance consistently poor?" If the individual has shown a more sudden change in behavior and in cognitive decline, then there is a possibility of depression (Siegel & Gershon, 1987).

Further observational information pertinent to the assessment of depression focuses on the overall disposition of the older person toward tasks and symptoms of the disease. Individuals with dementia tend to put effort into and derive pleasure from the accomplishment of tasks, but minimize symptoms of cognitive loss. In contrast, individuals with depression put forth minimal effort into the performance of tasks, but put great emphasis on symptoms of cognitive loss! The varying dispositions can be observed during day-to-day caregiving.

Finally, further assessment would include Geriatric Depression Scale (Yesavage & Brink, 1983). Individuals should be able to answer yes/no questions as determined in the assessment of Interactional Abilities. The scale consists of 30 questions requiring answers of yes or no (Figure 5.2).

The Geriatric Depression Scale is a reliable, valid measure of

1. Are you basically satisfied with your life? (no)
2. Have you dropped many of your activities and interests? (yes)
3. Do you feel that your life is empty? (yes)
4. Do you often get bored? (yes)
5. Are you hopeful about the future? (no)
6. Are you bothered by thoughts that you just cannot get out of your head? (yes)
7. Are you in good spirits most of the time? (no)
8. Are you afraid that something bad is going to happen to you? (yes)
9. Do you feel happy most of the time? (no)
10. Do you feel helpless? (yes)
11. Do you often get restless and fidgety? (yes)
12. Do you prefer to stay home at night, rather than go out and do new things? (yes)
13. Do you frequently worry about the future? (yes)
14. Do you feel that you have more problems with memory than most? (yes)
15. Do you think it is wonderful to be alive now? (no)
16. Do you often feel downhearted and blue? (yes)
17. Do you feel pretty worthless the way you are now? (yes)
18. Do you worry about the past? (yes)
19. Do you find life very exciting? (no)
20. Is it hard for you to get started on new projects? (yes)
21. Do you feel full of energy? (no)
22. Do you feel that your situation is hopeless? (yes)
23. Do you think that most persons are better off than you are? (yes)
24. Do you frequently get upset over little things? (yes)
25. Do you frequently feel like crying? (yes)
26. Do you have trouble concentrating? (yes)
27. Do you enjoy getting up in the morning? (no)
28. Do you prefer to avoid social gatherings? (yes)
29. Is it easy for you to make decisions? (no)
30. Is your mind as clear as it used to be? (no)

Note. From *Development & Validation of a Geriatric Depressions Screening Scale: A Preliminary Report.* By Yesavage, J. A. and Brink, T. L., 1983. *Journal of Psychiatric Research* 17:41. Copyright© 1983 Pergamon Press Inc. Reprinted with permission from Yesavage, J. A. and Brink, T. L.

Figure 5.2
The Geriatric Depression scale is a 30-item questionnaire that is used for the assessment of depression.

depression and originally consisted of 30 questions that are answered by "yes" or "no." It was developed from a larger questionnaire with 100 items. A score of over eight had about 90% sensitivity and 80% specificity in detecting depression in elderly patients.

NURSING ACTIONS

Ability Enhancing

When the ability to perceive pleasure is retained, as indicated by the presence of positive feeling states and the absence of depression, nursing actions which are ability enhancing are:

1. the determination and provision of pleasant activities;
2. the promotion of humor;
3. identification and validation of feelings, and attention to worries.

Teri and Logsdon (1991) contend that one of the most debilitating consequences of Alzheimer's disease is the individual's gradual loss of ability to perform activities that are rewarding and enjoyable. One way to determine which activities may be pleasurable is to complete the Pleasant Events Schedule (Teri & Logsdon, 1991). This schedule examines the frequency with which an individual undertakes an activity, the availability, and the enjoyability of the activity for the individual. Those activities that are enjoyable and available are then offered with the desired frequency indicated by the individual. If the individual is unable to provide this information, family members can be asked to complete the activities schedule.

Humor, and especially laughter, is believed to be ability-enhancing in relation to perceiving pleasure. It is believed that laughter stimulates the production of catecholamines (Peter & Dana, 1982), which may physiologically increase the ability to perceive pleasure. Ability-enhancing approaches recommended with respect to humor and laughter were discussed in the Social Abilities chapter.

Validation of the individual's perception, behaviors, and facial expressions acknowledges the importance of the older person's feelings to the nurse and reinforces their continued expression. Asking questions such as "Are you feeling sad or worried?" or offering feedback such as "you look happy today" creates opportunities for the individual to express feelings and for the nurse to intervene. A gentleman in our long-term care unit exhibited behavior that exemplified the value of exploration and validation. Mr. M. was described as disoriented, agitated, aggressive, and incontinent shortly after admission to the unit. Through nursing assessment, it was determined that the disorientation of Mr. M. was variable. There were times he was more oriented than others. The nurses decided to accept his behavior but listen to his concerns. A repeated "worry" concerned money and his son. The nurses contacted his son. It was learned that Mr. M.'s son was moving to another country and had been taking care of Mr. M.'s finances. The responsibility of Mr. M.'s finances was transferred to the financial department of the institution. Mr. M., his son and the facility's financial advisor together predetermined expenditures, and this provided reassurance to Mr. M. His behavior changed dramatically. He became responsive, calm, and continent. Furthermore, he was able to share his active sense of humor and repertoire of jokes.

NURSING ACTIONS

Ability Compensating

When the ability to perceive pleasure is absent, or depression exists, ability-compensating actions are:

1. the determination of previous life patterns in expressing feelings;
2. the provision of cognitive-behavioral strategies;
3. the encouragement of grief expression, through the establishment of trust and the communication of caring;
4. referral to psychiatry and monitoring of response to medication.

For those elders who have lost the ability to even respond to pleasure, it becomes critical to attend to behavioral changes and to learn their meaning. Behaviors such as agitation and angry out-bursts are indicative of feeling states. From Shomaker (1987), we understand that there is a continuity of previous life patterns re-lated to expression of emotion. Therefore, it would be helpful to ask family members to describe the person's previous life pattern re-lated to expressions of emotion. Also, ask the family about their own perception of what feelings might be affecting the person. When the basis of emotionally related behavior is understood, one's behavior is easily tolerated.

Cognitive–behavioral interventions for the treatment of de-pression in Alzheimer's patients have been described by Teri and Gallagher-Thompson (1991). Cognitive therapy challenges the negative perceptions of older persons with cognitive impairment to decrease distortions and to enable these individuals to generate more adaptive ways of viewing specific situations and events. Be-cause this requires a degree of cognitive ability and a commitment to do the homework involved in the therapy, it is suitable only for those with mild dementia. Behavioral interventions can be used alone for older persons with more advanced dementia, or in conjunc-tion with cognitive therapy with mild dementia . These approaches modify person–environment interactions by decreasing experiences of a negative or unpleasant nature. They include: the identification of stimuli or antecedents related to maladaptive responses such as withdrawal or agitation, identifying sources of complaints and mod-ifying these where possible, encouraging pleasant reminiscences and activities, and ensuring calm and accepting approaches by caregivers. Behavioral approaches are based on careful determina-tion of the older person's capabilities, and others evolve from col-laboration with psychology or psychiatry.

When the ability to perceive pleasure is lost, grief expression is encouraged. This consists of assisting the individual to express her feelings as able and appreciating nonverbal expressions of grief such as sighing and crying. This is preceded by the development of a sense of trust and the communication of caring through a consistent caregiver and planned time spent with the person on a regular basis.

A referral to psychiatry may be necessary for treatment of depression. When antidepressants are prescribed, monitor the older person's response to the medications by checking the vital signs, and observe for any signs of postural hypotension. Other important side effects include: anticholinergic changes, increased drowsiness, and increasing confusion. There are risks in prescribing antidepressants to the older-age population. A contrasting view is that of Reifer and Larson (1989) who found that attention and placebos were as effective as antidepressants in treating depression.

• CONCLUSION •

The abilities of older persons with dementia to interpret and respond to the world, to people, objects and events, and to perceive pleasure are affected by dementia. Careful attention to the assessment of an individual's interpretive abilities guides nursing care decisions that assist the individual to derive meaning from the external world, and to feel comfort with her own internal feeling states.

• *REFERENCES* •

Abrahams, J. P., & Camp, C. J. (1991, November). Maintenance and generalization of object naming training in anomia associated with degenerative dementia. Paper presented at The Gerontological Society of America Scientific Meeting, San Francisco, CA.

Akerlund, B. M., & Norberg, A. (1986). Group psychotherapy with demented patients. *Geriatric Nursing, 7*(2), 83–84.

Albert, M. S., Cohen, C., & Koff, E. (1991). Perception of affect in patients with dementia of the Alzheimer type. *Archives of Neurology, 48,* 791–795.

Arkin, S. M. (1991). Memory training in early Alzheimer's disease: An optimistic look at the field. *The American Journal of Alzheimer's Care and Related Disorders and Research, 6*(4), 17–25.

Brosgole, L., Kurucz, J., Plahovinsak, T. J., Sprotte, C., & Haveliwala, Y. A. (1983). Facial- and postural-affect recognition in senile elderly persons. *International Journal of Neuroscience, 22,* 37–46.

Carpenito, L. J. (1989). *Nursing diagnosis: Application to clinical Practice.* Philadelphia: J. B. Lippincott.

Cohen-Mansfield, J. (1986). Agitated behaviors in the elderly. *Journal of the American Geriatrics Society, 34,* 722–727.

Cummings, J. L., Miller, B., Hill, M. A., & Neshkes, R. (1987). Neuropsychiatric aspects of multi-infarct dementia and dementia of the Alzheimer type. *Archives of Neurology, 44,* 389–393.

Damasio, A. R., Damasio, H., & Van Hoesen, G. W. (1982). Prosopo-agnosia: Anatomic basis and behavioral mechanisms. *Neurology (NY), 32,* 331–341.

deLeon, M. J., Potegal, M., & Gurland, B. (1984). Wandering and parietal signs in senile dementia of Alzheimer's type. *Neuropsychobiology, 11,* 155–157.

Diesfeldt, H. F. A. (1990). Recognition memory for words and faces in primary degenerative dementia of the Alzheimer type and normal old age. *Journal of Clinical and Experimental Neuropsychology, 12,* 931–945.

Eslinger, P. J., & Benton, A. L. (1983). Visuoperceptual performances in aging and dementia: Clinical and theoretical implications. *Journal of Clinical Neuropsychology, 5,* 213–220.

Feil, N. (1992). Validation therapy with late onset and dementia populations. In G.M.M. Jones & B. Miesen (Eds.), *Care-giving in dementia: Research and applications.* (pp. 199–218.) New York: Tavistock/Routledge.

Förstl, H., Burns, A., Jacoby, R., & Levy, R. (1991). Neuroanatomical correlates of clinical misidentification and misperception in senile dementia of the Alzheimer type. *Journal of Clinical Psychiatry, 52,* 268–271.

Fromholt, P., & Larsen, S. F. (1991). Autobiographical memory in normal aging and primary degenerative dementia (dementia of Alzheimer type). *Journal of Gerontology, 46,* 85–91.

Gallo, J. J., Reichel, W., & Andersen, L. (1988). *Handbook of geriatric assessment.* Rockville, MD: Aspen.

Geiger, B. F. (1988). Cognitive intervention in Alzheimer's disease. *Journal of Rehabilitation, 54(3),* 21–24.

Gubrium, J. F., & Ksander, M. (1975). On multiple realities and reality orientation. *The Gerontologist, 15,* 142–145.

Gurland, B., & Toner, J. (1987). The epidemiology of the concurrence of depression and dementia. In H. Altman (Ed.), *Alzheimer's disease: Problems, prospects and perspectives* (pp. 45–57.) New York: Plenum.

Hoffman, S. B., Platt, C. A., Barry, K. E., & Hamill, L. A. (1985). When language fails: Nonverbal communication abilities of the demented. *Senile Dementia of the Alzheimer: Type, Neurology and Neurobiology, 18,* 49–64.

Issacs, B., & Kennie, K. T. (1973). The set test is an aid to dementia in old people. *British Journal of Psychiatry, 123,* 467–470.

Kane, R. L., Ouslander, J. G., & Abrass, I. B. (1989). *Essentials of clinical geriatrics* (2nd ed.). New York: McGraw-Hill.

Kopelman, M. D. (1989). Remote and autobiographical memory, temporal context memory and frontal atrophy in Korsakoff and Alzheimer patients. *Neuropsychologia, 27,* 437–460.

Kral, V. A. (1983). The relationship between senile dementia (Alzheimer type) and depression. *Canadian Journal of Psychiatry, 28,* 304–306.

Kurlycheck, R. T. (1983). Use of a digital alarm chronograph as a memory aid in early dementia. *Clinical Gerontologist, 1,* 93–94.

Kurucz, J., Feldmar, G., & Werner, W. (1979). Prosopo-affective agnosia associated with chronic organic brain syndrome. *Journal of the American Geriatrics Society, 27,* 91–95.

Martin, A., & Fedio, P. (1983). Word production and comprehension in Alzheimer's disease: The breakdown of semantic knowledge. *Brain and Language, 19,* 124–141.

Mattice, M., & Mitchell, G. J. (1990). Caring for confused elders. *Canadian Nurse, 86*(11), 16–18.

Miller, E. (1975). Impaired recall and the memory disturbance in presenile dementia. *British Journal of Social and Clinical Psychology, 14,* 73–79.

Mitchell-Pederson, L. (1990, September). The chief stranger. Presented at the annual conference of the Gerontological Nurses Association of British Columbia, Vancouver, B.C.

Morris, R., Wheatley, J., & Britton, P. (1983). Retrieval from long-term memory in senile dementia: Cued recall revisited. *British Journal of Clinical Psychology, 22,* 141–142.

Nebes, R. D., Boller, F., & Holland, A. (1986). Use of semantic context by patients with Alzheimer's disease. *Psychology and Aging, 1,* 261–269.

Peter, L. & Dana, B. (1982). *The laughter prescription: How to achieve health, happiness and peace of mind through humor.* New York: Ballantine Books.

Pryse-Phillips, W., & Murray, T. J. (1986). *Essential neurology* (3rd ed.). New York: Medical Examination Publishing Company.

Reifler, B. V., & Larson, E. (1989). Excess disability in dementia of the Alzheimer's type. In E. Light and B.D. Lebovitz (Eds.), *Alzheimer's disease treatment and family stress: Directions for research* (pp. 363–382). Rockville, MD: National Institute of Health.

Reisberg, B. (1983). Clinical presentation, diagnosis, and symptomatology of age-associated cognitive decline and Alzheimer's disease. In B. Reisberg (Ed.), *Alzheimer's disease: The standard reference* (pp. 173–187). New York: The Free Press.

Rosswurm, M. A. (1989). Assessment of perceptual processing deficits in persons with Alzheimer's disease. *Western Journal of Nursing Research, 11,* 458–468.

Ryden, M. B., & Knopman, D. (1989). Assess not assume: Measuring the morale of cognitively impairedelderly. *Journal of Gerontological Nursing, 15*(11), 27–32.

Sainsbury, R. S., & Coristine, M. (1986). Affective discrimination in moderately to severely demented patients. *Canadian Journal on Aging, 5,* 99–104.

Sheikh, J. I., & Yesavage, J. A. (1986). Geriatric Depression Scale (GDS): Recent evidence and development of a shorter version. In T.L. Brink (Ed.), *Clinical gerontology: A guide to assessment and intervention* (pp. 165–173). New York: Haworth.

Shomaker, D. (1987). Problematic behavior and the Alzheimer patient: Retrospection as a method of understanding and counselling. *The Gerontologist, 27,* 370–375.

Shulman, K., Shedletsky, B., & Silver, I. L. (1986). The challenge of clock drawing and cognitive function in the elderly. *International Journal of Geriatric Psychiatry, 1,* 135–140.

Siegal, B., & Gershon, S. (1987). Dementia, depression, and pseudodementia. In H. Altman (Ed.), *Alzheimer's disease: Problems, prospects and perspectives* (pp. 29–44). New York: Plenum.

Steele, C., Rovner, B., Chase, B., & Folstein, M. (1990). Psychiatric symptoms and nursing home placement of patients with Alzheimer's disease. *American Journal of Psychiatry, 147,* 1049–1051.

Teri, L., & Gallagher-Thompson, D. (1991). Cognitive-behavioral interventions for treatment of depression in Alzheimer's patients. *The Gerontologist, 31,* 413–416.

Teri, L., & Logsdon, R. G. (1991). Identifying pleasant activities for Alzheimer's disease patients: The Pleasant Events Schedule—AD. *The Gerontologist, 31,* 124–127.

Teri, L., Reifler, B. V., Veith, R. C., Barnes, R., White, E., McLean, P., & Raskind, M. (1991). Imipramine in the treatment of depressed Alzheimer's patients: Impact on cognition. *Journal of Gerontology, 46,* 372–377.

Wands, K., Merskey, D.M., Hachinski, V. C., Fisman, M., Fox, H., & Boniferro, M. (1990). A questionnaire investigation of anxiety and depression in early dementia. *Journal of the American Geriatrics Society, 38*(5), 535–538.

Wells, C. E., (1979) Pseudodementia. *American Journal of Psychiatry, 136,* 895.

Whiteley, A. M., & Warrington, E. K. (1977). Prosopo-agnosia: A clinical, psychological, and anatomical study of three patients. *Journal of Neurology, Neurosurgery, and Psychiatry, 40,* 395–403.

Wilson, R. S., Kaszniak, A. W., Bacon, L. D., Fox, J. H., & Kelly, M. P. (1982). Facial recognition memory in dementia. *Cortex, 18,* 329–336.

Wilson, R. S., Kaszniak, A. W., & Fox, J. H. (1981). Remote memory in senile dementia. *Cortex, 17,* 41–48.

Wilson, R. S., Kramer, R. L., Fox, J. H., & Kaszniak, A. W. (1983). Word frequency effect and recognition memory in dementia of the Alzheimer type. *Journal of Clinical Neuropsychology, 5,* 97–104.

Wragg, R. E., & Jeste, D. V. (1989). Overview of depression and psychosis in Alzheimer's disease. *American Journal of Psychiatry, 146,* 577–581.

Yesavage, J. A. (1982). Degree of dementia and improvement with memory training. *Clinical Gerontologist, 1,* 77–80.

Yesavage, J. A., Brink, T. L., Terence, L. R., Lum, O., Huang, V., Adey, M., & Leirer, V. O. (1983). The development and validation of a geriatric depression screening scale: A preliminary report. *Journal of Psychiatric Research, 17,* 37–49.

Zarit, S. H., Zarit, J. M., & Reever, K. E. (1982). Memory training for severe memory loss: Effects on senile dementia patients and their families. *The Gerontologist, 22,* 373–377.

SIX

CLOSING THOUGHTS

• THE VALUE OF A CONCEPTUAL AND RESEARCH-BASED PRACTICE •

This book began with an imaginative journey to portray how a progressive and irreversible cognitive impairment might change the world and the experiences of individuals. The journey served as an introduction to the multiple and discrete ways in which dementia affects older persons, and to the complexity of providing nursing care. Each chapter of the book described and discussed facets of dementia and specific related nursing care requirements. We believe that this knowledge, based on a conceptual model and a rigorous method of interpreting the research literature, is critical for nurses to be sensitive and responsive to the multiple needs of older persons with dementia.

At this time of fiscal restraint, nurses have a responsibility to convey both the complexity and benefits of providing knowledgeable and therapeutic care. A danger of the current preoccupation with limited resources in the provision of health care may be a gradual regression of caregiving practices to that of a custodial nature. Care and attention to the abilities of the individual is accorded little importance within the context of custodial care. There is widespread agreement that when a custodial approach prevails, support for the independence and dignity of people with dementia is sacrificed. As we have pointed out in the book, this creates tremendous potential for excess disability. It is only through a perspective like Enablement that continuity and quality of life can be preserved.

The Enablement perspective as presented in this book can serve as a beginning in articulating the ability-enhancing and compensating-caregiving approaches necessary for cognitively impaired older persons. This perspective can be used by gerontological nurses to counter any inappropriate reduction of resources allocated to this population. Present and continued work in this area can help to answer a number of valuable questions. Does the loss of extension abilities extend time for bathing? Does participation in self-bathing prolong the maintenance of extension abilities and prevent contractures, but require more intensive nursing care initially? Does the provision of relaxation and massage reduce episodes of agitation or anxiety, and hence, demands on caregivers' time? By systematically asking and answering questions such as these, gerontological nurses are able to convey the risks and/or benefits of custodial versus ability-enhancing care. We can then engage with other decisionmakers in determining appropriate resource allocation to the health care of cognitively impaired individuals.

A rigorously derived knowledge base can help us guide the development of policies and clinical practices. For example, gerontological nurses can take an advocacy role in (re)-designing workload measurement systems that better reflect the caregiving requirements of older people with dementia.

Gerontological nurses also have a responsibility to translate knowledge to family and other caregivers who are not conversant with current research. Many caregivers in long term care are non-professionals. Family members provide care to cognitively impaired individuals for many years before seeking admission of their relative to long-term care. Although kindness may be a primary motive in their caregiving, kindness without knowledge may inadvertently impose the risk of excess disability and greater caregiver burden.

In translating knowledge, the effect of the disease can be explained in terms of the older person's behaviors as observed by caregivers. The meaning of these behaviors in relation to threatened abilities can be described. Actions that preserve abilities or that compensate for their loss, and that are specific and feasible to implement, can be taught within the Enablement context. Many of the approaches suggested in this book may also provide enjoyment for both the older person and her caregivers. Explaining the value of activities such as throwing balls, sharing jokes, or singing and playing musical instruments may be revitalizing. It is also important to ask family and other caregivers about the actions they are using. Through trial and error, caregivers commonly find effective and enabling approaches. The Enablement knowledge base is then shared to affirm the soundness of the caregiver's actions.

• *FUTURE DIRECTIONS* •

More research about the effects of dementia is available, and we intend to continue to interpret it for the practice of nursing in the context of the Enablement perspective and the Content Methodology Process. We are planning a number of studies to evaluate the responsiveness of older persons with dementia to the ability-enhancing and ability-compensating approaches described in this book. We are also interested in the meaning of partial scores on components of the Abilities Assessment. We suspect that one interpretation of partial scores is that of impending excess disability. In this case, nursing approaches will be evaluated against the goal of achieving a positive change in the score on a follow-up assessment. It is our hope that other nurses will be inspired by the Enablement perspective, and will conduct intervention studies and share their interests and findings with us.

The use and application of the Enablement perspective need not be limited to the diseases of progressive dementia. There are other diseases, such as stroke and Parkinson's disease, which are experienced by older persons, and other content areas of nursing, such as mobility and continence, which can be studied. There are also other dimensions of the experience of dementia that can be examined for their impact on abilities and day-to-day living. Although we have discussed the importance of environment in the care of cognitively impaired older persons, we have not rigorously analyzed specific aspects of the environment in relation to the discrete abilities threatened. Aspects of the grief process that accompanies dementia, such as role change and loss, also affects an individual's abilities. These are content areas that can be developed in congruence with the Enablement perspective and the Content Methodology Process.

To end our book, we return to the imaginative journey. An implicit theme throughout this journey was a feeling of displacement and lack of connection with the persons and events encountered on the train. This was also exemplified in the remarks of the woman described in the Interpretive Abilities chapter, who found herself in a world of strangers—*"I live in a world of strangers and I am the chief stranger."* Through the Enablement perspective, and the promotion of retained abilities, the continuity of the familiar is ensured. The burden of the unfamiliar is decreased through compensation of lost abilities. Older persons who come to experience Alzheimer's dementia will find themselves on a journey. Let us practice nursing in such a way as to be perceived as fellow travelers who enhance the connectedness, the comfort, and the dignity of these older persons.

APPENDIX
ABILITIES ASSESSMENT

• *SELF-CARE ABILITIES* •

	Yes (1)	*No* (0)

1. *Voluntary Movements*

(a) *lips:* maintains relaxation of the lips when light pressure is applied in the form of a tongue blade or flexed finger moved along the lips

                                    Score ____ (1)

(b) *fingers:* maintains finger extension when the examiner stimulates the palm of the open hand with a finger

       (R) _____
       (L) _____

                                    Score ____ (2)

	Yes (1)	No (0)

(c) *arms:* passively extends the arm to some
extent after each of four times that the
examiner bends and extends the per-   (R) _____
son's arm   (L) _____

                                    Score ____ (2)
                              Subtotal ____ (5)
                                  (1. a–c)

2. *Spatial Orientation*
   (a) Right/Left Orientation
       Ask person to demonstrate awareness of left and right orienta-
       tion in simple (single) complex (in combination) or other (an-
       other person) levels:

	Yes (1)	No (0)

Single: (i) touch your right hand   ____   ____
            (ii) touch your left foot   ____   ____

Complex: (i) touch your right ear with
                 your left hand   ____   ____
            (ii) point to your left eye with
                 your right hand   ____   ____

*Other
Person:*   (i) touch my left hand   ____   ____
            (ii) touch my right hand   ____   ____
                                    Score   ____ (6)

	Yes (1)	No (0)

(b) Point of Origin
    Is able to return to room/home without
    assistance (i.e. finding own room)   ____   ____
                                    Score   ____ (1)
                              Subtotal ____ (7)
                                  (2. a–b)

3. *Purposeful movements*

(a) *Initiation and Follow-Through*

(i) Show 3 objects (pen, spoon, soap) ____ (3)
to the individual and ask him/her ____ (3)
to use them—if done correctly, ____ (3)
score for each correct. If done *incorrectly,* proceed to:

OR

(ii) Demonstrate the use of the objects ____ (2)
and ask the person to copy your ____ (2)
actions. Score 2 for each correct. If ____ (2)
done *incorrectly,* proceed to:

OR

(iii) Place the objects (one at a time) ____ (1)
in person's hand and ask person ____ (1)
to use each one. ____ (1)

Score ____ (9)

(b) *Simple Activity*

Individual performs 2 simple tasks in
ADL using "one" object.

(i) Instruct individual to comb hair:

	Yes (1)	No (0)
initiates activity	____	____
follows through activity by self	____	____
stops activity by self	____	____
sequences activity properly (i.e., in right order)	____	____

(ii) Instruct individual to drink from
a cup:

	Yes (1)	No (0)
initiates activity	____	____
follows through activity by self	____	____

	Yes (1)	No (0)
stops activity by self	____	____
sequences activity properly (i.e., in right order)	____	____
	Score ____ (10)	

(c) *Complex Activity*

Individual performs 2 complex tasks that require the use of more than one object, and switching from one activity to another.

(i) Instruct individual to wash hands using a washcloth and soap:

	Yes (1)	No (0)
initiates activity	____	____
follows through activity by self	____	____
stops activity by self	____	____
sequences activity properly (i.e., in right order)	____	____

(ii) Instruct individual to put on socks and shoes:

	Yes (1)	No (0)
initiates activity	____	____
follows through activity by self	____	____
stops activity by self	____	____
sequences activity properly (i.e., in right order)	____	____
	Score ____ (10)	
	Subtotal ____ (29)	
	(3. a–c)	

SELF-CARE ABILITIES SCORE

(a) Total score (add subtotals) = ____

(b) Total possible score = <u>41</u>

(c) % Score = $\dfrac{(a)}{(b)} \times 100$

%

· *SOCIAL ABILITIES* ·

Abilities

1. *To Give and Receive Attention*
    (a) greet person with "Hello", "Good morning", etc. Response is *one* of the following:
        - (i)   a verbal reply   ___ (4)
        - (ii) smile only   ___ (3)
        - (iii) eye contact only   ___ (2)
        - (iv   mutters   ___ (1)
        - (v)   no change in behavior to suggest response   ___ (0)

        Score   ___ (4)

    (b) initiate a handshake (i.e., offer your hand to the person). Response is *one* of the following:
        - (i)   grasps offered hand (self-initiated)   ___ (3)
        - (ii) other initiated (you take his/her hand)   ___ (2)
        - (iii) initiates letting go   ___ (1)
        - (iv) no response   ___ (0)

        Score   ___ (3)

    (c) individual's response to "how are you" is *one* of the following:
        - (i)   a verbal reply   ___ (3)
        - (ii) verbal but unclear   ___ (2)
        - (iii) nonverbal (eye gaze, nod, smile)   ___ (1)
        - (iv) no change in behavior to suggest response   ___ (0)

        Score   ___ (3)

(d) address individual by name and give your name. Response is *one* of the following:

  (i)   name repetition (repeats your name) or self-introduction ___ (4)
  (ii) facial response (nods, smiles, looks) ___ (3)
  (iii) body language response (leans toward) ___ (2)
  (iv) mumbles ___ (1)
  (v)   no response ___ (0)

                        Score   ___ (4)
                        Subtotal ___ (14)
                        (1. a–d)

2. *To Engage/Participate in Conversation*
   Initiate a topic of conversation with the individual. Response is *one* from topic and verbal, and any from nonverbal.

   (a) *Topic*
       stays on topic ___ (2)
       relates improbable events ___ (1)
       no response to topic ___ (0)
                        Score   ___ (2)

   (b) *Verbal*
       distinct verbal responses ___ (2)
       indistinct verbal response ___ (1)
       no verbal response ___ (0)
                        Score   ___ (2)

   (c) *Nonverbal*
       takes turns looks,   (1)
       listens or nods ___ (1)
       no response ___ (0)
                        Score   ___ (2)
                        Subtotal ___ (6)
                        (2. a–3)

3. *Humor Appreciation*

   (a) Inform individual that you have a cartoon you would like to show him. Show cartoon. Response is *one* of the following:

laughs out loud or makes relevant comments	____ (3)
laughs quietly	____ (2)
smiles	____ (1)
no response	____ (0)
Score	(3)

   (b) Inform individual that you have a joke you would like to tell him/her. Tell a *short* joke which is nonprejudicial and noncontroversial. Keep a straight face at the punch line. Example: "A kangaroo walked into a bar and asked the bartender for a beer. The bartender gave the kangaroo a beer and said 'That'll be 5 dollars.' Later the bartender returned and said 'We don't get many kangaroos in here.' The kangaroo said 'I'm not surprised, at these prices.'" Response is *one* of the following:

laughs at punch line or makes relevant comments	____ (3)
changes facial expression at the punch line	____ (2)
unexpected response at punch line (e.g., crying, anger, etc.)	____ (1)
no response	____ (0)
Score	____ (3)
Subtotal	____ (6)
(3. a–b)	

4. *Music Appreciation*

   (a) On a tape recorder, record player or radio, play some music (appropriate to his/her previous interests). Response is *any* of the following:

becomes quiet during music	____ (1)
sounds: singing, humming, relevant comments	____ (1)

body movement: taps feet or
hands, sways body, etc.   ____ (1)
no change in behavior to indicate
response   ____ (0)

Score	____ (3)
Subtotal	____ (3)

(4. a)

SOCIAL ABILITIES SCORE

(a) Total score (add subtotals) = ____

(b) Total possible score = $\underline{29}$

(c) % Score $= \dfrac{(a)}{(b)} \times 100$ [____ %]

• *INTERACTIONAL ABILITIES* •

1. *Comprehension Abilities*

Understanding of commands   Yes (1) No (0)

(i) *One-Part—self*

ask individual to follow four 1-part, (1 verb, 1 noun) commands relating to self: e.g.,

touch your nose   ____   ____

raise your arms   ____   ____

point to your feet   ____   ____

close your eyes   ____   ____

(ii) *One-Part—object*

ask individual to follow four, 1-part, (1 verb, 1 noun) commands relating to self: e.g.,

point to the ceiling   ____   ____

open the book   ____   ____

touch the chair   ____   ____

(iii)   *Two-Part—self*
   ask individual to follow three 2-part, (2 verbs, 2 nouns)
      commands relating to self: e.g.,
   stamp your feet and then close
      your eyes   ___ ___
   touch your cheek and pat your
      head   ___ ___
   blow through your lips and then
      point to your teeth   ___ ___

(iv)   *Two-Part—object*
   ask individual to follow three, 2-part commands relating
      to objects: e.g.,
   give me the pen, then point to
      the window   ___ ___
   touch the chair and point to the
      bed   ___ ___
   look at the floor and touch my
      ring   ___ ___

                                   Yes (1) No (0)

(v)   *Three-Part—Simple*
   ask individual to follow *two* simple (1 verb, 3 nouns)
      3-part commands: e.g.,
   point to your knees, then point
      to your head and then point to
      your stomach   ___ ___
   pick up the pen, pick up the cloth
      and then pick up the spoon   ___ ___

(vi)   *Three-Part—Complex*
   direct individual to follow *two* complete (3 verbs, 3
      nouns) 3-part commands: e.g.,
   point to my face, raise your
      arms, and clap your hands   ___ ___
   put your hands on the chair
      arms, slide your bottom for-
      ward, and stand on your feet   ___ ___
                            Score   ___ (18)

(b) *Yes/No Sentence Comprehension*

    (i)   Ask individual to respond yes or no to the following questions:

	Yes (1)	No (0)
Does Tuesday come after Thursday?	___	___
Is ice cream colder than coffee?	___	___
Do cars go faster than planes?	___	___
Is summer warmer than winter?	___	___
Score	___ (4)	

(c) *Reading Comprehension*

For the following, show the individual written commands of increasing complexity (1-part to 3-part commands). Each command should be on a separate page or card and be written large enough for the person to see. Present one at a time. Ask the individual to follow through on the command. Then ask the person to read the command aloud.

    (i)   *One-Part*

Ask individual to follow through on three 1-part commands. Ask the person to read the command aloud.

	Follow through (1)	Incorrect (0)	Read (1)	Incorrect (0)
e.g., point to the ceiling	___	___	___	___
touch my arm	___	___	___	___
hand me the pen	___	___	___	___

    (ii)   *Two-Part*

Repeat and score for three 2-part written commands.

	Follow through (1)	Incorrect (0)	Read (1)	Incorrect (0)
e.g., raise your arm(s) and close your eyes	___	___	___	___

	Follow through (1)	Incorrect (0)	Read (1)	Incorrect (0)
point to the ceiling and touch my arm	____	____	____	____
grap the arms of the chair and turn your head	____	____	____	____

(iii) *Three-Part*
repeat as in (a) and score for two 3-part written commands.

	Follow through (1)	**Incorrect (0)**	**Read (1)**	**Incorrect (0)**
e.g., point to the floor, touch the arm of the chair and then take my hand	____	____	____	____
put your hands on your knees, look at me and count to three	____	____	____	____

Score:
Follow through ____ (8) + Read ____ (8) = ____ (16)
Subtotal: ____ (38)
(1. a–c)

2. *Expression Abilities*
   (a) *Verbal object identification*
   Use four objects which are familiar and seen daily, e.g., pen, comb, fork, spoon, cup are held up and the person is asked to name the object. The person may name a related object, e.g., pen for pencil, glass for cup.

	Correct (2)	Related (1)	Incorrect (0)
	——	——	——
	——	——	——
	——	——	——
	——	——	——

Score   —— (8)

(b) *Word Retrieval*
    Completes the last word of four familiar
    sentences.

	Correct (2)	Related (1)	Incorrect (0)
e.g., The grass is — (green)	——	——	——
Ice is ———— (cold)	——	——	——
Violets are — (blue)	——	——	——
They fought like cats and —— (dogs)	——	——	——

Score   —— (8)

(c) *Description*
    Ask the individual to describe the room
    in which the assessment is taking place.

Scoring:

Description includes 4 or more objects (including floor,
    ceiling, walls) used in sentence form   —— (5)
Description includes 4 or more objects but sentences
    incomplete   —— (4)
Description includes less than 4 objects but they are correct—— (3)
Description includes less than 4 objects but they are
    incorrect   —— (2)
Verbal response attempted but no object words used   —— (1)
No response or verbal reaction   —— (0)

Score   —— (5)

(d) *Written Expression*

    (i)   Show the individual the object and ask individual to write
        its name e.g.; cup, pen, book

                              Yes (1) No (0)

                              ____   ____

                              ____   ____

                              ____   ____

    (ii)   Show the individual three familiar objects and ask in-
        dividual to write what these objects are used for, e.g., to
        drink, to write, to read

                              ____   ____

                              ____   ____

                              ____   ____

    (iii)   If score, is on i) and ii) but writing attempted and words
         not clear, give one point   ____ (1)

                          Score ____ (7)

                          Subtotal ____ (28)

                          (2. a–d)

INTERACTIONAL ABILITIES SCORE

(a) Total score achieved (add subtotals) = ____

(b) Total possible score = <u>41</u>

(c) % Score = $\dfrac{(a)}{(b)} \times 100$

                                               %

• *INTERPRETIVE ABILITIES* •

1. *Recognition*

                                    Yes   *No*

                                    (1)   (0)

(a) *Self-Recognition*

    (i)   identify self in mirror   ____   ____

	Yes (1)	No (0)

(ii)   ask person to read her/his own
name and then ask whose name it
is (i.e., what does this say Ms./Mr.
____ ? Who is that person?)   ____   ____

Score   (2)

(b) *Facial Affect Recognition*
Inform individual that you would like
him/her to tell you how the person in the
picture is feeling by the expression on
his/her face. Record description. If no
verbal description, ask individual to
choose if facial expression is sad, angry
or happy.

	Correct (1)	Not Correct No Reply(0)
(i) sad	____	____
(ii) angry	____	____
(iii) happy	____	____

Score ____ (3)

(c) *Object Recognition by Touch*

	Yes (1)	No (0)

(i)   Ask individual to close eyes and   ____   ____
identify 4 small objects placed in   ____   ____
hand, one at a time by touch   ____   ____
(e.g., comb, ring, key, spoon, or
fork).   ____   ____

(ii)   Ask individual to close eyes. Put large cup (e.g., Dixie
cup) in one hand and a small cup (e.g., medication cup) in
the other. Ask the individual to identify the hand holding
the larger cup.   ____   ____

Score ____ (5)

(d) *Recognition of Time*

	Yes (1)	No (0)

(i) *Clock*

Show the individual a drawing of a clock showing a specific on-the-hour time and ask the person to say what time is indicated on the clock. ____ ____

Show individual a drawing of a clock showing hour and minute time and ask the person to say what time is indicated on the clock. ____ ____

Score ____ (2)

	Yes (1)	No (0)

(ii) *Date*

Show individual a monthly calendar and ask to point out two dates. ____ ____

____ ____

	Yes (1)	No (0)

Point to *two* dates on a monthly calendar and ask individual to read these dates. ____ ____

____ ____

Score ____ (4)

Subtotal ____ (16)

2. *Recall*

   (a) Recall of familiar objects and places (F.A.C.T. test)
   Ask individual to recall as many fruits as possible. Repeat for animals, colors, and towns.

	3(8–10 items)	2(5–7)	1(1–4)	0(0)
F	____	____	____	____
A	____	____	____	____
C	____	____	____	____
T	____	____	____	____

   Score ____ (12)

   Subtotal ____ (12)

3. *Feeling States*
   (a) *Subjective*
   Inform the individual that you would like to talk with him/her about how he/she has been feeling in the last week. When asking the following questions, it may be necessary to preface with probes (e.g., "Do you have feelings now of ___ ?" or "Have you ever had feelings of ___ ?")

(i)	sadness (no)	____
(ii)	anxiety (no)	____
(iii)	happiness (yes)	____
(iv)	worry (no)	____
(v)	contentment (yes)	____
(vi)	boredom (no)	____

Score 1 if answers given are as shown.

Score   ____ (6)
Subtotal   ____ (6)

   (b) *Depression*
   Suspect depression if the individual expresses no to numbers iii, & v, and yes to numbers i, ii, iv, and vi. Return to pages 126 & 127 of the text for direction. Depression is another level of assessment and not part of the "Abilities Assessment."

INTERPRETIVE ABILITIES SCORE
(a) Total score achieved (add subtotals) =

____

(b) Total possible score = ____

(c) % Score = $\frac{(a)}{(b)} \times 100$ ☐ %

Author Index

SUBJECT INDEX

COMFORTING THE CONFUSED
Strategies for Managing Dementia

Stephanie B. Hoffman, PhD, and
Constance A. Platt

"Hoffman and Platt have undertaken the task of seeking to limit pain and suffering of the dementia victims and their caregivers. They offer effective, research-based, practical guidelines for communicating with dementia patients at all levels of disability. They offer strategies for responding to depression, hostility, wandering and other behaviors often accompanying dementia."

—From the Foreword by **Eric Pfeiffer,** MD
University of South Florida

1991 225pp 0-8261-7850-2 *hardcover*

TREATMENTS FOR THE ALZHEIMER PATIENT

Lissy F. Jarvik, MD, PhD, and
Carol H. Winograd, MD, Editors

"...offering readers multiple strategies for treating the disease...emphasizes that Alzheimer's disease affects not only the patient but also the family and caretakers. Perspectives from physicians, family members and sociologists are well documented, and practical advice on handling difficult conditions commonly associated with Alzheimer's disease is provided....I recommend it to anyone involved in the care of elderly persons."

—**American Family Physician**

1988 288pp 0-8261-6000-X *hardcover*